Control
of Appetite

CURRENT CONCEPTS IN NUTRITION

Myron Winick, Editor

Institute of Human Nutrition
Columbia University College of Physicians and Surgeons

CONTROL
OF APPETITE

Edited by

MYRON WINICK

Institute of Human Nutrition
College of Physicians and Surgeons
Columbia University
New York, New York

A WILEY-INTERSCIENCE PUBLICATION

JOHN WILEY & SONS, INC.

New York • Chichester • Brisbane • Toronto • Singapore

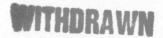

Library of Congress Cataloging-in-Publication Data

Control of appetite.

  (Current concepts in nutrition, ISSN 0090-0443;
v. 16)
  "A Wiley-Interscience publication."
  Includes bibliographies and index.
  1. Appetite. 2. Appetite disorders. 3. Eating
disorders. I. Winick, Myron. II. Series.
[DNLM: 1. Appetite. 2. Appetite—Disorders—
physiopathology. 3. Appetite Regulation. 4. Feeding
Behavior. 5. Neuroregulators—physiology.
W1 CU788AS v.11 / WI 102 C764]
QP136.C66 1988   616.3′9   87-28005
ISBN 0-471-63743-2

Printed in the United States of America

10 9 8 7 6 5 4 3 2 1

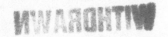

Preface

This volume covers an area which brings together the research of psychologists, nutritionists, neuroscientists, and pharmacologists in an attempt to integrate current knowledge about how appetite is controlled. The ten chapters include a detailed discussion of both central and peripheral neurotransmitters and how they are related to appetite control. In addition, the most up-to-date pharmacological research involving drugs which can affect central transmitters is discussed. Finally, there are several chapters dealing with clinical situations in which appetite control is altered. These include pregnancy and lactation, cancer, anorexia nervosa, and bulimia. During pregnancy and lactation, appetite increases as more calories are consumed. In patients with cancers of various types, anorexia may develop. Patients with anorexia nervosa and bulimia show an abnormal regulation of food intake. All of these conditions can supply clues as to how normal food intake is regulated and what goes wrong under certain conditions.

Appetite is also involved in the complex process of feeding behavior which encompasses not only biologic and pathologic control but also psychologic control. Two chapters deal with psychologic factors in appetite regulation and in the use of food.

This volume, therefore, while highlighting work in several different disciplines, has focused on a current problem in nutrition, appetite control, in a comprehensive manner. The reader should come away with an up-to-date knowledge of the "state of the art" of this complex subject.

MYRON WINICK, M.D.

New York, New York
August 1987

Contents

1

Animal Models of Appetitive Behavior: Interaction of Nutritional Factors and Drug Seeking Behavior

ROBIN B. KANAREK, Ph.D.,
and ROBIN MARKS-KAUFMAN, Ph.D.
Department of Psychology, Tufts University, Medford, Massachusetts, and
Institute of Human Nutrition, Columbia University, New York, New York

Research using experimental animals has laid the foundation for much of our knowledge about appetitive behavior. To provide some background about the role this research has played in our understanding of appetitive behaviors, we shall discuss three related issues. First we shall present a brief overview of animal models of appetitive behavior. Second, we shall discuss carbohydrate induced obesity in animals, a model of experimental obesity that we have been investigating for a number of years. Finally, although this book is primarily concerned with feeding as an appetitive behavior, it is clear that food is not the only substance that humans and animals "self-administer." Both our own species and a number of experimental animals self-administer a variety of psychoactive agents. During the past several years, increasing attention has been paid to the interaction of nutritional variables and drug self-administration. This research is discussed in the final section of this chapter.

The research reported in this chapter was supported in part by NIH Grant AM-31653 to R.B.K. and Grant DA-03940 to R.M-K.

1

ANIMAL MODELS OF APPETITIVE BEHAVIOR

Research with experimental animals has provided important information about both the normal control of food intake and abnormalities that can occur in feeding behavior (e.g., anorexia nervosa, bulimia, and obesity). It has been suggested that the alterations in food intake observed in anorexia nervosa and bulimia may be mimicked in experimental animals by damage to portions of the central nervous system (e.g., lateral hypothalamus) (1,2). However, careful analysis of the deficits in feeding behavior found in brain-damaged animals and those found in people with anorexia nervosa and bulimia indicate that the conditions are not comparable (1). Thus, at present, there are no good animal models of either of these eating disorders (1,3).

Animal Models of Obesity

Genetic Obesity. In contrast to the situation with anorexia nervosa and bulimia, a variety of animal models of obesity exist (4). In 1953, Mayer (5) divided the factors that can lead to obesity in experimental animals into three major categories: genetic, traumatic, and environmental. As shown in Table 1-1, there are a number of experimental animals in which obesity results primarily as a function of genetic factors (6–9). Genetically obese rodents have been divided according to mode of inheritance into single gene dominant strains (e.g., yellow obese mouse; adipose mouse), single gene recessive strains (e.g., ob/ob mouse; Zucker rat), and polygenic strains (e.g., New Zealand obese mouse; spiny mouse; sand rat). Among these single gene recessive models, the greatest amount of attention has been paid to the ob/ob mouse and the Zucker fatty rat. Some of the basic characteristics of these animals include hyperphagia, increased feed efficiency (weight gained per kilocalories consumed), adipocyte hypertrophy and hyperplasia, hyperinsulinimia, and decreased diet induced thermogenesis (4,6–10).

Table 1-1.   Selected Animal Models of Experimental Obesity

Genetic Models

Single gene, dominant   ·
      Yellow obese mouse
      Adipose mouse
Single gene, recessive
      ob/ob mouse
      db/db mouse
      Zucker fatty rat (fa/fa)
Polygenic, spontaneously obese
      New Zealand obese mouse
      Japanese mouse
      Wellesley mouse
      NH mouse
Polygenic, obesity prone
      Osborne-Mendel rat
      Sand rat (*Psammomys obesus*)
      Spiny mouse (*Acomys cahirinus*)

Traumatic Models

Neural
      Ventromedial hypothalamic lesions
      Paraventricular lesions
      Midbrain lesions
Endocrine
      Chronic insulin administration
      Ovariectomy
      Chronic glucocorticoid treatment

Environmental Models

Physical restraint
Stress induced
Nutritional
      Force feeding
      Meal feeding
      High fat diets
      Cafeteria diets
      High sugar diets

Traumatic Obesity. Models of traumatic obesity include animals that overeat and suffer the consequences of obesity as a result of factors such as damage to the central nervous system (CNS), manipulations of the endocrine system, and pharmacological treatments (see Table 1-1). Of these models, animals whose obesity results from the destruction of the portion of the CNS known as the ventromedial hypothalamus (VMH) have dominated research for over four decades (6,11,12). Obesity in VMH lesioned animals is associated with hyperphagia, increased feed efficiency, dietary finickiness, adipocyte hypertrophy, hyperinsulinimia, and decreased diet induced thermogenesis (6,12).

Within the last several years, it has been recognized that damage to other portions of the CNS, including the paraventricular nucleus (PVN) (13,14) and midbrain area (15,16) also can lead to increases in food intake, body weight, and adiposity in experimental animals. The obesity produced by damage to the PVN and midbrain area is similar in many respects to that produced by VMH lesions. The effects of these manipulations, however, are not identical. For example, midbrain lesions, in contrast to VMH lesions, result in selective deposition of fat in the intrascapular region, an area with high brown fat content (15).

Environmental Obesity. Environmental factors that can lead to increases in body weight and adiposity include physical restraint (17) and stressful stimulation, such as tail pinch (18). Over the past decade, environmental models in which dietary factors are associated with the development of obesity have caught the attention of many researchers (for reviews see (19–21)). These models are particularly attractive because they may mirror the human condition especially closely. In modern society, people are constantly exposed to many different appetizing and highly caloric foods. This situation often is associated with unwise food choices, increased food intake, and weight gain. Like humans, animals are susceptible to the obesity promoting effects of certain foods, and may become obese when offered diets high in fat or sugar, or when given a variety of palatable foods (so called cafeteria or supermarket diets).

Early research on diet induced obesity used high fat diets (22–27). In these and subsequent experiments, it was observed that normal animals typically consume less of a high fat diet than of a low fat diet. However, although animals fed a calorically dense high fat diet decrease food intake, they usually consume more calories per day than animals fed a less calorically dense low fat diet. Depending on the strain of the experimental animals, increases in caloric intake in animals fed high fat diets can range from 5% to over 25% (26,28–31). Although obesity in animals fed high fat diets is related to an increase in caloric consumption, an enhancement of feed efficiency also contributes to the observed increases in body weight (32–37).

Obesity in animals fed high fat diets is associated with increases in both size and number of fat cells (adipocytes) (32,38–40). Evidence suggests that diet induced increases in adipose tissue mass depend on a fixed order of events. Animals on high fat diets first show an increase in fat cell size. Once a critical cell size is reached, the formation of new fat cells is triggered (38). While diet induced hyperplasia is now a well-documented phenomenon, specific morphologic changes produced by high fat diets may be site specific. The growth of different fat pads probably follows the same general pattern in response to high fat feeding. However, the critical cell size that triggers hyperplasia may vary for different fat depots (33,38). Although increases in fat cell number seem to occur only after a period of cell hypertrophy, it is important to note that once diet induced cell proliferation occurs, it is not reversible (38).

Besides inducing morphologic changes in adipose tissue depots, high fat diets produce a number of metabolic alterations. Hyperinsulinemia is a common correlate of many forms of obesity, and may be observed in rats made obese with high fat diets (40,41). High fat diets also produce significant elevations in circulating levels of free fatty acids, triglycerides, cholesterol, and glycerol (40,41).

Nutritional obesity also can be produced in experimental animals by feeding them a diet that has been called by various investigators a "cafeteria," "supermarket," or "junk food" diet (42–50). This model of obesity was first described by Dr. Anthony Sclafani and colleagues (42,43). These investigators observed that obesity could be produced by offering rats a variety of palatable foods normally marketed for human consumption (e.g., chocolate chip cookies, marshmallows, salami, cheese, peanut butter, and sweetened condensed milk). Rats offered these foods increased daily caloric intake and rapidly gained weight relative to animals fed only a standard laboratory diet (42,43). The excess weight gain of adult rats fed cafeteria diets is due primarily to an increase in adipose tissue stores (42–44,51) associated with increases in both fat cell size and number (51).

The potential parallels with the human situation have made cafeteria induced obesity a particularly compelling model to study. However, several factors may detract from its overall usefulness as a model of obesity. First, with a cafeteria diet it is difficult to measure daily energy intake accurately. In most experiments using cafeteria diets, the energy content of food items is only estimated from published food tables. Further, rats are notorious for spilling and mixing cafeteria items, making precise determinations of total energy intake problematic (52). Second, the exact composition of cafeteria diets varies substantially among laboratories. Moreover, each animal displays individual preferences for food (53) and each cafeteria item has a different macronutrient profile. Therefore, the nutrient composition of the diet is not constant from animal to animal. This variation makes it impossible to determine the effects of a particular nutrient on weight gain and adiposity. Finally, cafeteria diets differ from standard laboratory diets in a number of ways, including nutritional quality, sensory aspects, variety of items offered, and postabsorptive consequences. The importance of each of these factors to the development of hyperphagia and obesity with "cafeteria" diets currently is under debate (48,53,54).

Another nutritional method that has been used to produce obesity in experimental animals is feeding diets high in simple carbohydrates. Early research investigating the role of carbohydrates in the production of obesity concentrated on evaluating the effects of different types of carbohydrates (i.e., simple vs. complex) on food intake, body weight gain, and adiposity. In these experiments, one group of animals received a diet containing a complex carbohydrate (e.g., corn starch), while a second group was fed a diet in which the complex carbohydrate was replaced by a simple sugar (e.g., sucrose). In reviewing these early studies, no clear pattern of results emerges with respect to the effects of different carbohydrates on energy intake. Energy intakes of rats fed high sucrose diets have been reported to be greater than (55–57), equivalent to (58–63), or less than (64,65) those of animals given a high starch diet. Similar inconsistencies are evident when the effects of different carbohydrates on body weight and adiposity are reviewed. Although rats consuming high sucrose diets typically exhibit increased body weight or adiposity or both relative to animals consuming high starch diets (55,56,64,66,67) this is not universally the case (58,59,61,63,64,68–70). The studies cited above differed in a number of ways, including the strain, age, and sex of the animals used, diet composition, and the length of the experiment. All of these factors may contribute to the conflicting results observed when animals are fed high sucrose diets.

In contrast to the conflicting findings on the effects of single high sucrose diets on the development of obesity, recent research has demonstrated that obesity can reliably be produced by giving rats a simultaneous choice of a nutritionally complete diet and a palatable carbohydrate solution (71–79). Most experiments using this choice have used sucrose for the carbohydrate solution. However, solutions made from other sugars, such as fructose and maltose (20,73), and polysaccharides, such as Polycose (80), also can promote obesity in experimental animals.

The majority of studies investigating the effects of carbohydrate solutions on the development of obesity have offered rats a choice of Purina Rodent Chow (Ralson Purina Co.) and a 32% sucrose solution (20,71–76,79–81). Rats given this choice eat only 40% to 50% as much Purina Chow as animals given only the Chow diet. However, these rats avidly consume the sucrose solution, resulting in a total daily energy intake that is typically 15% to 20% greater than that of animals not given the sugar solution (20,71,73–77,79).

Over time, the small but reliable increment in caloric intake observed in rats fed Purina Chow and a sucrose solution translates into substantial increases in body weight gain and adiposity (20,71–77,79). In adult animals, significant elevations in body weight and adipose tissue mass are seen within 2 to 3 weeks after this dietary regime is begun (20,72–77). In comparison, when

weanling rats are given Chow and a sucrose solution, no differences in body weight are noted between these animals and those
given only Chow until the animals are approximately 70 days of
age (71). However, indirect measures of adiposity indicate that differences in body fat deposition between the two groups of rats
occur as early as 42 days of age (71). Additionally, direct determinations of body composition demonstrated that while rats given a
sucrose solution and Chow do not weigh more at 70 days of age,
they do have significantly more body fat than animals fed only
Chow (71). Work by Faust and colleagues (38) has documented that
the increase in body fat seen in adult rats drinking a sucrose solution is the result of increases in both fat cell size and number.

In adult animals, the elevation in body weight and adiposity
observed in rats drinking sucrose solutions is associated with not
only an increase in caloric intake, but also an increase in feed
efficiency (72,73,80). Indeed, increased weight gain can occur in
rats consuming a sucrose solution without a concomitant elevation
in total caloric intake (72,80).

Obesity in rats drinking a sucrose solution is associated with
many of the metabolic changes frequently observed in human
obesity (82,83). Animals fed sucrose show hyperglycemia and
impaired glucose tolerance after an oral glucose load (73). Additionally, hyperinsulinemia frequently accompanies consumption
(79, Kanarek, Marks-Kaufman, and Orthen-Gambill, unpublished
results). Rats given sucrose also show increases in plasma triglycer-
ide levels (73) and elevations in blood pressure (84,85) relative to
animals fed only a standard laboratory diet. Finally, in recent
work, we observed that sucrose consumption makes rats more susceptible to the actions of the diabetogenic drug streptozotocin
(STZ) (Kanarek and Hirsch, unpublished results). After STZ
administration, rats that had been drinking a sucrose solution had
higher mortality rates than their counterparts not given sucrose.
Additionally, rats that had received sucrose before STZ injections
had higher fasting plasma glucose levels and showed greater elevations in glucose values after an oral glucose load than animals not
exposed to the sugar.

SUCROSE AND REINFORCEMENT

Given the detrimental consequences of sucrose intake, it may be surprising that when given a choice, animals continue to consume excessive amounts of the sugar. However, much evidence supports the idea that sucrose, or the sensory quality associated with sugar ingestion (palatable sweet taste), is reinforcing. This evidence includes demonstrations that in short term taste tests, rats overwhelmingly prefer sucrose to water and moreover, prefer high concentrations of sucrose to lower concentrations (86,87). Further, nondeprived rats will perform a variety of operant responses to obtain small amounts of sugar solutions or nonnutritive sweet tasting saccharin solutions (88–90). Data on the compelling nature of sweet tastes come from experiments in which rats were given access to food and either a sucrose or saccharin solution for a limited time each day (1 hour). During this time, rats avidly drank the sweet tasting solutions and failed to consume sufficient amounts of food to maintain their body weight (91,92). Despite continued weight loss, rats did not alter their pattern of behavior and died of starvation when maintained on this feeding schedule for extended periods of time.

For humans, preferences for sweet tastes appear to be unlearned and occur as early as several hours after birth (93–95). Recent work has demonstrated that in adults, consumption of palatable high carbohydrate foods can lead to feelings of relaxation, warmth, and contentment (96).

It has been hypothesized that sucrose may have addictive properties. Although it is certainly too early to draw this conclusion, research that we and others have been conducting implies that there may be an interaction between sucrose consumption and addictive psychoactive drugs.

NUTRITIONAL VARIABLES AND DRUG SELF-ADMINISTRATION

Work begun in the early 1960s showed that psychoactive drugs with abuse liability in humans, such as heroin and amphetamine, are readily self-administered by experimental animals (97–101). In contrast, psychoactive agents without abuse liability in humans are not self-administered by animals.

One drug that has been studied extensively by using self-administration procedures is morphine (102–106). Several years ago, we began to investigate the interaction between nutritional variables and oral self-administration of morphine in rats. In these studies, self-administration was established by replacing the animals' water with a 0.8 mg/ml morphine solution. Hence, to maintain fluid balance, rats had to drink the morphine solution. Initially, the bitter taste of the morphine solution inhibited fluid intake. However, within 3 to 4 days, 70% to 80% of the rats began to drink the drug solution. As previously reported (103–106), considerable variation was observed in daily oral morphine intake. However, this variation was not random. Rats that drank the morphine solution exhibited three to four day cycles in fluid intake. Over time, these animals became physically dependent on morphine. Animals developed a preference for the morphine solution and demonstrated symptoms of withdrawal when the drug was removed or when they were injected with a narcotic antagonist (naloxone).

Effects of Food Deprivation on Drug Self-Administration

Research had shown that animals' patterns of drug administration can be modified by altering access to food. Carroll and Meisch (107–115) reported that food deprivation increases self-administration of a variety of psychoactive drugs. For example, rats that were deprived of food to 75% of their free-feeding body weight drank twice as much of a 5 µg/ml solution of the synthetic opioid etonitazene as nondeprived animals. In contrast, similarly deprived animals that drank water exhibited a 50% reduction in fluid intake relative to nondeprived animals (108). As shown in Table 1–2, similar increases in drug intake have been observed in several species with different methods of drug administration and different classes of drugs (116–120,137–139).

As a result of the work by Carroll and Meisch (107–115), we examined the effects of food deprivation on oral morphine self-

Table 1-2. Food-Deprivation Induced Increases in Drug Self-Administration

Drug	Food Deprivation Schedule	Increase in Drug Intake	Reference
Rats			
D-amphetamine (iv)	80% free-feeding body weight	2 fold	(118)
Phetermine (iv)	80% free-feeding body weight	10 fold	(137)
Etonitazine (oral)	75% free-feeding body weight	2 fold	(109, 110)
Etonitazine (iv)	8 g food/day	2 fold	(138)
Cocaine (iv)	8 g food/day	2 fold	(138)
Phencyclidine (iv)	8 g food/day	2 fold	(138)
Ethanol (oral)	80% free-feeding body weight	2–3 fold	(117)
Heroin (iv)	80% free-feeding body weight	2–3 fold	(139)
Rhesus Monkeys			
Phencyclidine (oral)	75 g food/day	2–4 fold	(111)
D-amphetamine (oral)	85% free-feeding body weight	dose dependent[a]	(113)
Ketamine (oral)	85% free-feeding body weight	dose dependent[a]	(113)

[a]Food deprivation increased drug reinforced behavior; however, at higher concentrations of the drug the difference between responding in food satiated and food deprived conditions was attenuated.

administration. Rats were divided into three groups. The first group (N = 8) received water, the second group (N = 10) had water replaced with a 0.8% morphine sulfate solution, and the third group (N = 10) had water replaced with a 0.5% quinine solution. This last group was used to control for any effects of the bitter taste of the morphine solution. After a 40 day period of exposure to the drug solutions and ad libitum access to food, half of the animals in each group were reduced to 80% of their free-feeding weight by limiting food intake to 8 to 10 g per day.

Rats given the morphine solution initially decreased fluid intake relative to animals given water. Within a week, the majority of the animals began to consume the morphine solution and showed patterns of intake typical of rats orally administering morphine; that is, fluid intakes varied across a three to four day period. Food intakes of rats given morphine also varied from day to day and in general, were correlated with intake of the morphine solution. This cyclical pattern of fluid and food intake was not due to the bitter taste of the solution. Rats drinking the quinine solution decreased fluid consumption relative to animals given water, but did not show variations in daily fluid intake.

Rats that drank the morphine solution also showed alterations in diurnal patterns of fluid and food intake. Rats are normally nocturnal, consuming the majority of their food and fluid at night. In contrast, when the rats were given morphine, the proportion of food and fluid they consumed at night varied substantially on a day to day basis. For example, an individual animal might consume over 80% of its food and fluid at night on one day, and under 20% on the next. In comparison, animals that drank either water or the quinine solution consistently consumed 85% to 95% of their fluid and food at night.

Food deprivation led to substantial increases in morphine drinking (Fig. 1-1). In contrast, food deprivation resulted in decreases in both water and quinine intake (Fig. 1-2). One explanation for this finding is that food deprivation in some way alters the metabolic consequences of morphine intake. Another possibility is that the removal of one reinforcing substance (i.e., food), augments the intake of another reinforcing substance (i.e., morphine). To test this possibility, we conducted several experiments investigating the effects of another substance with reinforcing properties (sucrose) on oral morphine intake.

Interaction of Sucrose and Morphine Self-Administration

In our first experiment we found that sucrose had a profound effect on drug taking behavior. Twelve adult Sprague-Dawley rats

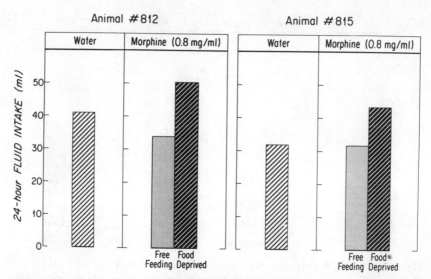

Figure 1-1. Twenty-four hour fluid intakes for two rats that were given a 0.8 mg/ml morphine sulfate solution as their sole source of fluid. The left hand panel for each animal represents water intake during a seven day predrug period. Daily morphine intake for each animal was averaged for the 40 day period when animals had ad lib access to food (free-feeding) and for the 16 day period when food was restricted to 8 to 10 g/day (food deprived).

initially received ad libitum access to ground Purina Chow, granulated sucrose, and water. On the seventh day of the study, water was replaced with either a 0.5 mg/ml morphine solution or a 0.8 mg/ml morphine solution. Ten days later, granulated sucrose was removed from all animals.

Figure 1-3 represents mean fluid intake for the rats in each group. These data also are very representative of the pattern of fluid intake shown by individual animals. All rats decreased fluid intake when water was replaced with a morphine solution. In both groups, removal of sucrose led to an increase in morphine consumption. When sucrose was available, five of the six rats given the 0.8 mg/ml morphine solution lost weight. Removal of sugar resulted in an increase in body weight. Although rats drinking the 0.5 mg/ml morphine solution gained weight when sucrose was present, they showed an increased rate of weight gain when sucrose was removed.

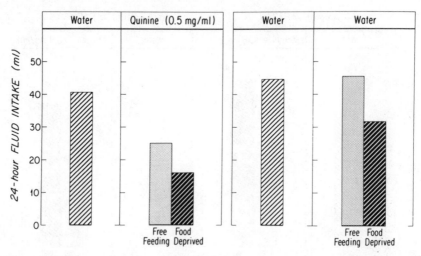

Figure 1-2. Twenty-four hour fluid intakes for one rat that received a 0.5 mg/ml quinine solution and for one rat that received water as their sole source of fluid. The left hand panel for each animal represents water intake during a seven day predrug period. Daily fluid intakes for each animal were averaged for the 40 day period when animals had ad lib access to food (free-feeding) and for the 16 day period when food was restricted to 8 to 10 g/day (food deprived).

   The results of this experiment provided preliminary evidence of an interaction between sucrose availability and oral morphine self-administration. The removal of sucrose led to an immediate increase in morphine intake. To assess the relation between sucrose and drug administration more fully, it was necessary to determine if the converse was true. That is, would the return of sucrose lead to a decrease in morphine intake? Two experiments were performed to answer this question.

   In our second experiment, all rats initially received ground Purina Chow, granulated sucrose, and water. On the seventh day of the study, water was replaced with a 0.8 mg/ml morphine solution for eight animals. The remaining six rats continued to receive water. Sucrose was removed from all animals six days later and returned after an additional 13 days.

   Only three of the eight rats given granulated sucrose and the morphine solution drank sufficient fluid to maintain body weight.

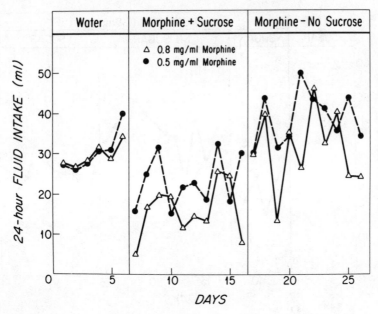

Figure 1-3. Mean daily fluid intake for rats given either a 0.8 mg/ml or a 0.5 mg/ml morphine sulfate solution. The left hand panel presents mean daily water intake during the six day predrug period. The middle panel presents daily drug intake when the animals had granulated sucrose and Purina Chow as nutrient sources. The right panel presents daily drug intake when granulated sucrose was removed.

The remaining five animals failed to drink the morphine solution and lost substantial amounts of weight. In the three rats that drank the morphine solution, a very distinctive pattern of intake was observed. As shown in Figure 1-4, which represents fluid intake for one of the animals that drank the morphine solution, fluid intake decreased when water was replaced with the morphine solution. Removing sucrose led to an immediate increase in morphine intake. When sucrose was again presented on day 25 of the study, morphine intake immediately was reduced. For the six animals that received water throughout the experiment, sucrose availability had no effect on fluid intake.

The results of this experiment again indicated a relation be-

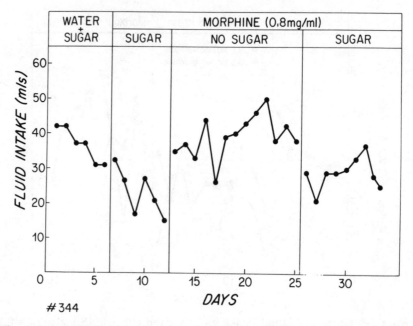

Figure 1–4. Daily fluid intake for an individual rat given a 0.8 mg/ml morphine sulfate solution as its sole source of fluid. The left hand panel presents daily water intake during the six day predrug period. For the next six days, this animal received granulated sucrose and Purina Chow as nutrient sources and the morphine solution as its fluid source. Granulated sucrose was then removed and was returned 13 days later.

tween sucrose availability and oral self-administration of morphine. Only 37% of the rats given sucrose and Purina Chow drank the drug solution. In contrast, in other experiments in which sucrose was not available, 60% to 80% of animals consumed the morphine solution. These data suggest that the availability of sucrose inhibits morphine self-administration. Additionally, sucrose altered drug taking behavior in animals that did drink the morphine solution. Animals consistently drank less of the morphine solution when sucrose was available than when the sugar was not available.

In our next study, we altered our procedure to obtain more rats that would drink the morphine solution. Rats were given brief pe-

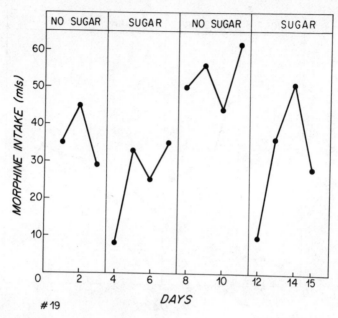

Figure 1-5. Daily morphine intake for an individual rat given a 0.8 mg/ml morphine solution as its sole source of fluid. Periods in which only Purina Chow was available were alternated with periods when both Purina Chow and granulated sucrose were available as nutrient sources.

riods of access to granulated sucrose (three to four days) alternated with periods when the sugar was not available. In addition, some animals began the experiment with access to only Purina Chow while others began with access to both Purina Chow and sucrose. With this procedure, over 80% of the rats orally self-administered morphine. As shown in Figures 1–5 and 1–6, very consistent patterns of intake again were observed, with animals drinking less of the morphine solution when given sucrose than when given only Purina Chow.

Recent work by Caroll and Boe (121) examining the effects of a glucose-saccharin solution on intravenous administration of etonitazene, a synthetic opioid, also demonstrates that the presence of a palatable sugar solution can mediate opioid intake. When rats

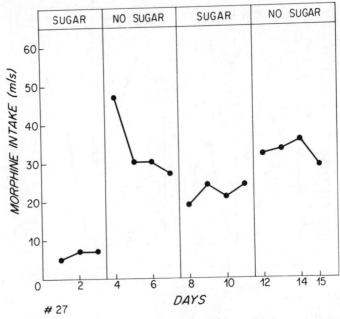

Figure 1-6. Daily morphine intake for an individual rat given a 0.8 mg/ml morphine solution as its sole source of fluid. This animal began the experiement with access to both Purina Chow and granulated sucrose.

were deprived of the sugar solution they showed small but reliable reductions in etonitazene self-administration.

There are at least two possible explanations for the interaction between sucrose availability and morphine consumption. First, sucrose may be producing its effect by acting on endogenous opioid systems. Data to support this possibility come from research examining the effects of sucrose consumption on opiate receptor binding. Opiate receptor binding in whole brain was increased in both genetically obese mice (ob/ob) and their lean littermates that had consumed Purina Chow and sucrose for four weeks when compared to binding in animals that had consumed only Purina Chow (122). Similar increases in opiate receptor binding were observed in weanling rats given access to sucrose for a three week period (122). The increase in binding was a function of an increase in binding affinity rather than an increase in receptor number.

Further evidence that the relation between sucrose and morphine may be mediated by the endogenous opioid system comes from research by Dum and colleagues (123,124), indicating that access to palatable foods that contain sucrose leads to increased release and breakdown of hypothalamic beta-endorphin in rats. Analogous findings in humans were reported by Getto and colleagues (125), who found that oral administration of a glucose solution increased plasma immunoreactive beta-endorphin levels in lean and obese subjects.

Research examining the effects of palatable sweet tasting solutions on opioid induced analgesia contributes indirect support for an interaction between sugar and the endogenous opioid system. In 1956, Davis and colleagues (126), using the tail flick test, observed that in rats glucose potentiated and prolonged the analgesic action of morphine. More recently, Leiblich (127), looking at the effects of highly palatable solutions on opioid analgesia, suggested that chronically elevated intake of a saccharin solution caused changes in the behavior of rats that were consistent with elevated endogenous opioid levels.

Finally, in a recent study, Fantino and colleagues (128) reported that the opioid antagonist naltrexone selectively reduced preference for sucrose in humans. In this experiment, nonobese subjects were asked to rate on a pleasure–displeasure scale sucrose and salty solutions as well as alimentary and nonalimentary odors. The effects of an intragastric glucose load (vs. water load) and naltrexone (vs. placebo) on the affective responses of subjects to the gustatory and olfactory stimuli were tested. Relative to the control conditions, both the glucose load and naltrexone produced a significant decrease in the subjects' liking for the sweet tasting solution. Naltrexone had minimal effects on subjects' affective responses to alimentary odors and no effect on responses to either the salty stimuli or nonalimentary odors. Fantino and colleagues concluded that naltrexone may produce its effect on sucrose preference by acting on the endogenous opioid system.

Although a specific association between sugar and opiates may exist, this relation also could represent a more general interaction between reinforcing substances. Sucrose availability has been found to alter not only morphine intake but also intake of other psychoactive drugs. For example, Lester and Greenberg (129) noted that when sucrose was made available to rats previously accustomed to drinking alcohol, animals decreased their alcohol intake to zero. Removal of sucrose led to an increase in alcohol consumption. More recently, Samson and colleagues (130) reported that rats showed a decreased response for alcohol when sucrose was concurrently available. Along similar lines, Carroll (131) observed that rhesus monkeys orally self-administered less phencyclidine (angel dust) when a palatable saccharin solution was available than when the solution was not available.

The preceding information suggests that in animals an inverse relation between intake of palatable sweet tasting substances and at least certain psychoactive agents may exist. Limited data indicate that a similar relation may exist in humans. First, studies on the dietary intake of alcoholics have revealed that alcoholics consumed significantly less sugar than nonalcoholic subjects. Further, Yung and colleagues (132), working in an alcoholism treatment program, noted that people who stayed sober for more than 30 days consumed significantly more sucrose and more overall carbohydrates than people who did not remain sober for the 30 days. Finally, investigators (133–136) recently have hypothesized an inverse relation between nicotine intake and the consumption of sweet tasting foods. In a number of experiments using both experimental animals and humans, it has been observed that nicotine administration is accompanied by decreased consumption of sweet foods. Conversely, cessation of nicotine intake results in increased sweet food consumption (133–136).

A relationship between diet and drug self-administration may have important implications for (1) the basic understanding of drug-seeking behavior and (2) the clinical treatment of drug abuse. Manipulations that decrease rate of drug self-administration have obvious relevance for treatment. Classically, rate of drug administration has been reduced by either behavioral measures, such as punishment, or pharmacologic means, such as methadone. Diet may be a more benign approach to dealing with this problem.

REFERENCES

1. S. F. Leibowitz, in P. L. Darby, P. E. Garfinkel, D. M. Garner, and D. V. Coscina, Eds., *Anorexia Nervosa, Recent Developments in Research*, Alan R. Liss, New York, 1983, pp. 221–229.

2. G. F. M. Russell, S. A. Checkley, and P. H. Robinson, in M. O. Carruba and J. E. Blundell, Eds., *Pharmacology of Eating Disorders: Theoretical and Clinical Developments*, Raven Press, New York, 1986, pp. 151–167.

3. N. Mrosovsky, in P. L. Darby, P. E. Garfinkel, D. M. Garner, and D. V. Coscina, Eds., *Anorexia Nervosa, Recent Developments in Research*, Alan R. Liss, New York, 1983, pp. 199–206.

4. A. Sclafani, *Int. J. Obes.*, **8**, 491 (1984).

5. J. Mayer, *Physiol. Rev.*, **33**, 472 (1953).

6. G. A. Gray and D. A. York, *Physiol. Rev.*, **59**, 809 (1979).

7. F. Contaldo, in L. A. Cioffi, W. P. T. James, and T. B. Van Itallie, Eds., *The Body Weight Regulatory System: Normal and Disturbed Mechanisms*, Raven Press, New York, 1981, pp. 237–242.

8. M. F. W. Festing, Ed., *Animal Models of Obesity*, Macmillan, London, 1979.

9. L. Herberg and D. L. Coleman, *Metabolism*, **26**, 59 (1977).

10. J. Himms-Hagen, *Ann. Rev. Nutr.*, **5**, 69 (1985).

11. S. P. Grossman, in L. A. Cioffi, W. P. T. James, and T. B. Van Itallie, Eds., *The Body Weight Regulatory System: Normal and Disturbed Mechanisms*, Raven Press, New York, 1981, pp. 11–17.

12. T. L. Powley, *Psychol. Rev.*, **84**, 89 (1977).

13. S. F. Leibowitz, N. J. Hammer, and K. Chang, *Physiol. Behav.*, **27**, 1031 (1981).

14. A. Sclafani and P. F. Aravich, *Am. J. Physiol.*, **244**, R686 (1983).

15. M. Box, R. Bascom, and G. J. Mogenson, *Behav. Neural Biol.*, **26**, 330 (1979).

16. L. Hernandez and B. G. Hoebel, *Brain Res.*, **245**, 327 (1982).

17. D. J. Ingle, *Proc. Soc. Exp. Biol. Med.*, **72**, 604 (1949).

18. N. E. Rowland and S. M. Antelman, *Science*, **191**, 310 (1976).

19. A. Sclafani, in A. J. Stunkard, Ed., *Obesity*, Saunders, Philadelphia, 1980, pp. 166–181.

20. R. B. Kanarek and E. Hirsch, *Fed. Proc.*, **36**, 154 (1977).

21. R. B. Kanarek and N. Orthen-Gambill, in Beyden, Ed., *Comparative Animal Nutrition*, Vol. 6, in press.

22. O. Mickelsen, O. Takahashi, and C. Craig, *J. Nutr.*, **57**, 541 (1955).

23. P. F. Fenton and C. J. Carr, *J. Nutr.*, **45**, 225 (1951).

24. R. Schemmel, O. Mickelsen, and L. Fisher, *J. Nutr.*, **103**, 477 (1973).

25. R. Schemmel, O. Mickelsen, and J. L. Gill, *J. Nutr.*, **100**, 1041 (1970).

26. R. Schemmel, O. Mickelsen, and U. Mostosky, *Anat. Rec.*, **166**, 437 (1970).

27. R. Schemmel, O. Mickelsen, and Z. Tolgay, *Am. J. Physiol.*, **216**, 373 (1969).

28. H. J. Carlisle and E. Stellar, *J. Comp. Physiol. Psychol.*, **69**, 107 (1969).

29. J. D. Corbit and E. Stellar, *J. Comp. Physiol. Psychol.*, **58**, 63 (1964).

30. J. Kirtland and M. I. Gurr, *Br. J. Nutr.*, **39**, 19 (1978).

31. L. B. Oscai, *Am. J. Physiol.*, **242**, R212 (1982).

32. L. Herberg, W. Doppen, E. Major, and F. A. Gries, *Lipid Res.*, **15**, 580 (1974).

33. K. C. Jen, M. R. C. Greenwood, and J. A. Brasel, *Physiol. Behav.*, **27**, 161–166 (1981).

34. L. B. Oscai, M. M. Brown, and W. C. Miller, *Growth*, **48**, 415 (1984).

35. J. M. Slattery and R. M. Potter, *Appetite*, **6**, 133 (1985).

36. G. N. Wade, *Physiol. Behav.*, **29**, 701 (1982).

37. J. D. Wood and J. T. Reid, *Br. J. Nutr.*, **34**, 15 (1975).

38. I. M. Faust, P. R. Johnson, J. S. Stern, and J. Hirsch, *Am. J. Physiol.*, **235**, E279 (1978).

39. B. J. Klyde and J. Hirsch, *J. Lipid Res.*, **20**, 705 (1979).

40. J. Triscari, C. Nauss-Karol, B. E. Levin, and A. C. Sullivan, *Metabolism*, **34**, 580 (1985).

41. B. E. Levin, A. Finnegan, J. Triscari, and A. C. Sullivan, *Am. J. Physiol.*, **248**, R717, (1984).

42. A. Sclafani and D. Springer, *Physiol. Behav.*, **17**, 461–471 (1976).

43. A. Sclafani and A. N. Gorman, *Physiol. Behav.*, **18**, 1021 (1977).

44. B. J. Rolls and E. A. Rowe, *Physiol. Behav.*, **23**, 241 (1979).

45. B. J. Rolls, E. A. Rowe, and R. C. Turner, *J. Physiol.*, **298**, 415 (1980).

46. E. A. Rowe and B. J. Rolls, *Physiol. Behav.*, **28**, (1982).

47. N. J. Rothwell, M. E. Saville, and M. J. Stock, *J. Nutr.*, **112**, 1515 (1982).

48. B. J. Rolls, V. Duijvenvoorde, and E. A. Rowe, *Physiol. Behav.*, **31**, 21 (1983).

49. P. J. Rogers and J. E. Blundell, *Neurosci. Biobehav. Rev.*, **8**, 441 (1984).

50. P. J. Rogers, *Physiol. Behav.*, **35**, 493 (1985).

51. D. Walks, M. Lavau, E. Presta, M-U. Yang, and P. Bjorntorp, *Am. J. Clin. Nutr.*, **37**, 387 (1983).

52. G. R. Hervey and G. Tobin, *Clin. Sci.*, **64**, 7 (1983).

53. M. Naim, J. G. Brand, M. R. Kare, and R. G. Carpenter, *J. Nutr.*, **115**, 1447 (1985).

54. J. Louis-Sylvestre, I. Giachetti, and J. LeMagnen, *Physiol. Behav.*, **32**, 901 (1984).

55. M. W. Marshall, M. Womack, H. E. Hildebrand, and M. E. Munson, *Proc. Soc. Exp. Biol. Med.*, **132**, 227 (1969).

56. S. Reiser and J. Hallfrisch, *J. Nutr.*, **107**, 147 (1977).

57. M. Suzuki, Y. Satoh, and N. Hashiba, *J. Nutr. Sci. Vitaminol.*, **29**, 663 (1983).

58. S. Al-Nagdy, D. Miller, and J. Yudkin, *Nutr. Metabol.*, **12**, 193 (1970).

59. A. Dulloo, O. Eisa, D. Miller, and J. Yudkin, *Am. J. Clin. Nutr.*, **42**, 214 (1985).

60. J. Hallfrisch, F. Lazar, and S. Reiser, *Am. J. Clin. Nutr.*, **32**, 787 (1979).

61. S. S. Kang, K. R. Bruckdorfer, and J. Yudkin, *Nutr. Metabol.*, **23**, 301 (1979).

62. D. J. Naismith and I. A. Rana, *Nutr. Metabol.*, **16**, (1974).

63. G. M. Reaven, T. R. Risser, Y-D. Chen, and E. P. Reaven, *J. Lipid Res.*, **20**, 371, (1979).

64. R. Allen and J. Leahy, *Br. J. Nutr.*, **20**, 339 (1966).

65. S. Reiser, O. Michaelis, J. Putney, and J. Hallfrisch, *J. Nutr.*, **105**, 894 (1975).

66. M. W. Marshall, H. E. Hildebrand, J. L. Dupond, and M. Womack, *J. Nutr.,* **69,** 371 (1959).

67. C. Berdanier, R. Tobin, and V. DeVore, *J. Nutr.,* **109,** 261 (1979).

68. J. Hallfrisch, L. Cohen, and S. Reiser, *J. Nutr.,* **111,** 531 (1981).

69. L. Dalderup and W. Visser, *Nature,* **222,** 1050 (1969).

70. H. Laube, C. Wojcikowski, H. Schatz, and E. F. Pfeiffer, *Horm. Metab. Res.,* **10,** 192 (1978).

71. R. B. Kanarek and R. Marks-Kaufman, *Physiol. Behav.,* **23,** 881 (1979).

72. W. Hill, T. Castonguay, and G. Collier, *Physiol. Behav.* **24,** 756 (1980).

73. R. B. Kanarek and N. Orthen-Gambill, *J. Nutr.,* **112,** 1546 (1982).

74. E. Kirsch, E. Ball, and L. Godkin, *Physiol. Behav.,* **29,** 253 (1982).

75. E. Hirsch, C. Dubose, and H. Jacobs, *Physiol. Behav.,* **28,** 819 (1982).

76. E. Hirsch and M. Walsh, *Physiol. Behav.,* **28,** 129 (1982).

77. S. Rattigan and M. G. Clark, *J. Nutr.,* **114,** 1971 (1984).

78. S. Muto and C. Miyahara, *Br. J. Nutr.,* **28,** 327 (1972).

79. J. Granneman and G. Wade, *Metabolism,* **32,** 202 (1983).

80. A. Sclafani and S. Xenakis, *Physiol. Behav.,* **32,** 169 (1984).

81. A. Sclafani and S. Xenakis, *Life Sci.,* **34,** 1253 (1984).

82. A. A. Rimm and P. L. White, in G. A. Bray, Ed., *Obesity in America,* U.S. Department of Health, Education, and Welfare, NIH Publication No. 79-359, 1979, pp. 103-124.

83. L. B. Salans, in G. A. Bray, Ed., *Obesity in America,* U. S. Department of Health, Education, and Welfare, NIH Publication No. 79-359, 1979, pp. 69-94.

84. R. D. Bunag, T. Tomita, and S. Sasaki, *Hypertension,* **5,** 218 (1983).

85. J. B. Young and L. Landsberg, *Metabolism,* **30,** 421 (1981).

86. P. T. Young and E. H. Shuford, Jr., *J. Comp. Physiol. Psychol.,* **48,** 114 (1955).

87. G. Collier and R. Bolles, *J. Comp. Physiol. Psychol.,* **65,** 379 (1968).

88. N. Guttman, *J. Exp. Psychol.,* **46,** 213 (1953).

89. J. Ganchrow and G. L. Fisher, *Psychol. Rep.,* **22,** 503 (1968).

90. F. D. Sheffield and T. B. Roby, *J. Comp. Physiol. Psychol.,* **43,** 471 (1950).

91. L. W. Hamilton, *J. Comp. Physiol. Psychol.,* **77,** 59 (1971).

92. A. Sclafani, *Physiol. Behav.,* **11,** 595 (1973).

93. J. A. Desor, O. Maller, and R. E. Turner, *J. Comp. Physiol. Psychol.,* **84,** 496 (1973).

94. J. A. Desor, O. Maller, and L. S. Greene, in J. M. Weiffenbach, Ed., *Taste and Development, The Genesis of Sweet Preference,* DHEW No. 77-1068, Washington, DC, 1977, pp. 161-172.

95. J. E. Steiner, J. M. Weiffenbach, Ed., *Taste and Development, The Genesis of Sweet Preference,* DHEW No. 77-1068, Washington, DC, 1977, pp. 173-187.

96. A. J. Hill, L. D. Magson, and J. E. Blundell, *Appetite,* **5,** 361 (1984).

97. G. A. Deneau, T. Yanagita, and M. H. Seever, *Psychopharmacologia,* **16,** 30 (1969).

98. C. R. Schuster and T. Thompson, *Ann. Rev. Pharmacol.,* **9,** 483 (1969).

99. C. E. Johanson, in D. E. Blackman and D. J. Sanger, Eds., *Contemporary Research in Behavioral Pharmacology,* Plenum, New York, 1978, pp. 325-390.

100. R. Pickens, R. A. Meisch, and T. Thompson, in L. L. Iversen, S. D. Iversen, and S. H.

Snyder, Eds., *Handbook of Psychopharmacology*, Vol. *12, Drugs of Abuse*, Plenum, New York, 1978, pp. 1–38.

101. C. E. Johanson and C. R. Schuster, in N. K. Mello, Ed., *Advances in Substance Abuse: Behavioral and Biological Research*, Vol. *2*, JAI Press, Greenwich, CT, 1982, pp. 219–297.

102. J. R. Weeks, *Science*, **138**, 143 (1962).

103. R. Marks-Kaufman and M. J. Lewis, *Addict. Behav.*, **9**, 235 (1984).

104. K. A. Khavari and M. E. Risner, *Psychopharmacologia*, **30**, 291 (1973).

105. I. P. Stolerman and R. Kumar, *Psychopharmacologia*, **17**, 137–150 (1970).

106. D. E. McMillan, J. D. Leander, T. W. Wilson, S. C. Wallace, T. Fix, S. Redding, and R. Turk, *J. Pharmacol. Exp. Ther.*, **196**, 269 (1976).

107. M. E. Carroll and R. A. Meisch, in T. Thompson, P. Dews, and J. E. Barrett, Eds., *Advances in Behavioral Pharmacology*, Vol. *4*, Academic Press, New York, 1984, pp. 47–88.

108. M. E. Carroll, C. P. France, and R. A. Meisch, *Science*, **205**, 319 (1979).

109. M. E. Carroll and R. A. Meisch, *Pharmacol. Biochem. Behav.*, **10**, 155 (1979).

110. M. E. Carroll and R. A. Meisch, *Psychopharmacology*, **68**, 121 (1980).

111. M. E. Carroll and R. A. Meisch, *J. Pharmacol. Exp. Ther.*, **214**, 339 (1980).

112. M. E. Carroll and R. A. Meisch, *Psychopharmacology*, **74**, 197 (1981).

113. M. E. Carroll and D. C. Stotz, *J. Pharmacol. Exp. Ther.*, **227**, 28 (1983).

114. M. E. Carroll, D. C. Stotz, D. J. Kliner, and R. A. Meisch, *Pharmacol. Biochem. Behav.*, **20**, 145 (1984).

115. M. E. Carroll, M. C. Pederson, and R. G. Harrison, *Pharmacol. Biochem. Behav.*, **24**, 1095 (1986).

116. R. A. Meisch and T. Thompson, *Psychopharmacologia*, **28**, 171 (1973).

117. R. A. Meisch and T. Thompson, *Pharmacol. Biochem. Behav.*, **2**, 589 (1974).

118. R. N. Takahashi, G. Singer, and T. P. S. Oei, *Pharmacol. Biochem. Behav.*, **9**, (1978).

119. M. Papasava, T. P. S. Oei, and G. Singer, *Pharmac. Biochem. Behav.*, **15**, 485 (1981).

120. M. Papasava and G. Singer, *Psychopharmacology*, **85**, 419 (1985).

121. M. E. Carroll and I. N. Boe, *Pharmacol. Biochem. Behav.*, **17**, 563 (1982).

122. R. Marks-Kaufman, M. Hamm, and G. F. Barbato, *Fed. Proc.* **44**, 424 (1985).

123. J. Dum, C. Gramsch, and A. Herz, *Pharmacol. Biochem. Behav.*, **18**, 443 (1983).

124. J. Dum and A. Herz, *Pharmacol. Biochem. Behav.*, **21**, 259 (1984).

125. C. J. Getto, D. T. Fullerton, and I. H. Carlson, *Appetite*, **5**, 327 (1984).

126. W. M. Davis, T. S. Miya, and L. D. Edwards, *J. Am. Pharmaceut. Assoc.*, **45**, 60 (1956).

127. I. Lieblich, E. Cohen, J. R. Ganchrow, E. M. Blass, and T. Bergman, *Science*, **221**, 871 (1983).

128. M. Fantino, J. Hosotte, and M. Apfelbaum, *Am. J. Physiol.*, **251**, R91 (1986).

129. D. Lester and L. A. Greenberg, *Quart. J. Stud. Alchol.*, **13**, 553 (1952).

130. H. H. Samson, T. A. Roehrs, and G. A. Tolliver, *Pharmacol. Biochem. Behav.*, **17**, 333 (1982).

131. M. Carroll, *J. Exper. Anal. Behav.*, **43**, 131 (1985).

132. L. Yung, E. Gordis, and J. Holt, *Drug Alcoh. Depend.*, **12**, 355 (1983).

133. N. E. Grunberg, *Addict. Behav.*, **7**, 317 (1982).

134. N. E. Grunberg, D. J. Bowen, and D. E. Morse, *Psychopharmacology*, **83**, 93 (1984).

135. N. E. Grunberg and D. E. Morse, *J. App. Soc. Psychol.*, **14**, 310 (1984).

136. N. E. Grunberg, D. J. Bowen, V. A. Maycock, and S. M. Nespor, *Psychopharmacology*, **87**, 198 (1985).

137. M. Papasava, G. Singer, and C. L. Papasava, *Psychopharmacology*, **85**, 410 (1985).

138. M. E. Carroll, C. P. France, and R. A. Meisch, *J. Phamacol. Exp. Ther.*, **217**, 241 (1981).

139. T. P. S. Oei, G. Singer, D. Jefferys, W. Lang, and A. Latiff, in F. C. Colpaert and J. A. Rosecrans, Eds., *Stimulus Properties of Drugs: Ten Years of Progress*, North Holland Elsevier, Amsterdam, 1978, pp. 506–516.

2

Neurotransmitters, Control of Appetite, and Obesity

RICHARD J. WURTMAN, M.D.
Department of Applied Biological Sciences and Clinical Research Center,
Massachusetts Institute of Technology, Cambridge, Massachusetts

Any complex set of behaviors—like deciding what and when to eat—must involve a very large number of neurons and many different neurotransmitters. The problem confronting the neuroscientist interested in control of appetite is not to catalogue all of these neurotransmitters but to identify the important ones—the ones released by neurons that have a unique function, perhaps of sensing the need to eat calories or particular nutrients, or of integrating this information with external sensory cues, or of deciding that eating should stop. If the strategy used to identify such neurotransmitters is too broad, all such compounds tested will probably be shown to have some effect on the appetite, but nothing will have been learned by this demonstration, except that ultimately every neuron in the brain is connected to every other neuron through neurotransmitters.

The strategy that we propose (and use) involves determining which transmitters, if any, are *themselves* affected by eating. Our studies, discussed below, and those of many other investigators provide evidence that brain serotonin is special, in that its own synthesis and release are enhanced by some foods, suppressed by others, and unchanged by yet others, *depending on their nutrient contents.* Transmitters are also affected by *not* eating, in a complex manner that can provide the brain with information about how much time has passed since the person last ate. These special properties allow serotonin-releasing neurons to occupy a central place in the control of one kind of appetite—that for eating appropriate proportions of proteins and carbohydrates—and also to affect appetite in general. The rest of this chapter describes these properties and their implications, especially for the very common form of obesity associated with "carbohydrate craving," which is typified by a vast intake of carbohydrates as snacks (but not at meals). It will also be seen, however, that these special properties of serotonin neurons exact a price: They may allow food consumption to affect other behaviors that happen to involve serotonin (e.g., sleepiness, sensitivity to environmental stimuli), and, conversely, may allow mood disturbances to override appetite control mechanisms, and cause the person to eat inappropriately.

Of course it can be prophesized that other brain neurotransmitters besides serotonin will turn out to have special and important roles in controlling the appetite. This chapter describes strategies that may be useful for identifying them, by looking for the neurotransmitters whose dynamics are themselves affected by eating. Several good candidates (that will not be discussed here further) are already known to exist, for example, acetylcholine and the catecholamines. The rates at which these compounds are liberated from physiologically active, frequently firing neurons are increased after treatments that raise brain levels of their precursors, choline and tyrosine. The involvement of these neurotransmitters in appetite regulation, however, remains highly uncertain, since few real foods exist that might be predicted to raise brain tyrosine, and little if any evidence is available that the increases in acetylcholine or catecholamine release caused by giving pure choline or tyrosine affect the appetite. For now, the neurotransmitter about which most can be said in relation to appetite regulation is serotonin.

EFFECTS OF CARBOHYDRATES ON BRAIN SEROTONIN

For the brain to be able to regulate eating, it must have access to signals about what has been eaten. This information cannot be limited to the sensory properties of the food—how it tastes or smells, or its apparent bulk—since two equally bulky (or tasty) foods can have very different caloric values and nutrient contents. Rather, the signals must relate to the *metabolic consequences* of having eaten the food, and must be capable of varying in proportion to whichever aspects of the food are being regulated, principally its caloric values and its contents of one or more macronutrients (proteins, carbohydrates, fats). Presumably, a food or meal should produce chemical changes in the brain, the nature and duration of which vary with the meal's nutrient contents and its size. And included among these neurochemical responses should be changes in the release of specific chemicals, the neurotransmitters, which the brain uses to carry instructions from one neuron to another.

Foods can indeed cause chemical changes in the brain (1–5). Moreover, these chemical changes apparently participate both in the normal regulation of food intake and in the pathophysiological processes that operate in some patients with obesity. Consumption of a *carbohydrate* rich meal rapidly increases the rate at which certain brain neurons produce and release their neurotransmitter serotonin (2); this signal then acts to diminish the likelihood that the person will consume carbohydrates in the next meal or snack, and to increase the likelihood of protein consumption (6,7). A *protein* rich meal has opposite effects. It tends to suppress the synthesis and release of serotonin (3), making the person more likely to eat carbohydrate (and less likely to eat protein) during his next meal.

Dietary *fat* has not yet been shown to have any consistent effects on brain neurotransmitters; moreover, currently available evidence provides little support for the view that the fat contents of meals are independently regulated (or that, as has been suggested, the brain senses the size or fullness of peripheral fat depots). However dietary fat can influence a meal's effect on the brain by *indirect* mechanisms. For example, it can diminish the rate at which the food is digested and absorbed, thus prolonging the effect of its carbohydrates or proteins on brain neurotransmitter synthesis.

The biochemical mechanisms through which dietary carbohydrates and proteins affect brain serotonin (and, under special circumstances, brain catecholamines (5,8)) involve the secretion of insulin and the effects of this hormone on plasma levels of most of the amino acids. The insulin secreted after a carbohydrate meal or snack profoundly depresses plasma levels of most large, neutral amino acids (LNAA), (e.g., leucine, isoleucine, and valine, and, to a lesser extent, tyrosine and phenylalanine); however, it has little or no effect on plasma tryptophan (9,10). As a consequence, it *raises* the "plasma tryptophan ratio" (the ratio of the tryptophan concentration to the summed concentrations of the other LNAA), thereby enhancing tryptophan's ability to be carried across the blood–brain barrier (by a transport macromolecule that is unsaturated with tryptophan, and that also transports the other LNAA, competitively (11)). The resulting increase in brain tryptophan levels enhances the saturation of the enzyme tryptophan hydroxylase and thereby accelerates the synthesis of serotonin. Dietary proteins have the opposite effect because, even though they contain some tryptophan (about 1%), and thus raise plasma tryptophan levels (10), they contain, proportionately, far greater amounts of the other LNAA, and thus lower the plasma tryptophan ratio. (The effect on brain serotonin of any meal or snack will also, of course, depend on how many hours have elapsed since the subject last ate, and on what he then ate: A carbohydrate rich snack will have only minor effects on the plasma tryptophan ratio in someone who is still digesting a large protein rich meal.)

BRAIN SEROTONIN AND NUTRIENT SELECTION

That the food-induced changes in brain serotonin are involved in subsequent food selection has been demonstrated in a variety of ways. For example, if rats are allowed to choose concurrently from among foods of differing nutrient contents (e.g., one food pan containing a 75% carbohydrate, 20% protein meal, and another containing a 25% carbohydrate, 20% protein food), it is observed that the number of grams of each food that they consume remains more or less constant from day to day among animals. Administration of drugs thought to enhance serotonin mediated neurotransmission will cause the animals to eat less of the carbohydrate rich food without having much effect on the consumption of the other diet (6,7). (It does not seem to be important whether the carbohydrate used in the diets happens to be sweet (12): nonsweet starches increase brain serotonin levels as well as sucrose and dextrose do, and are abjured by animals that have received serotoninergic drugs.) This selective effect of serotoninergic drugs on carbohydrate consumption differentiates these compounds from amphetamine-like compounds: Rats receiving the latter agents and given access to a single test meal will consume less of the meal, regardless of its nutrient contents. In contrast, the serotoninergic drugs will suppress consumption of the test meal only if it is relatively rich in carbohydrates (13). Presumably, the drugs modify eating behavior by "fooling the brain" into thinking that the animal is in the process of digesting a carbohydrate rich meal or snack. This hypothesis is affirmed by showing that giving rats a carbohydrate "snack" an hour before allowing them to choose between two test foods (for "dinner") has the same effect on nutrient choice as giving them a serotoninergic drug, that is, it causes them to eat less carbohydrate for "dinner" (without affecting the total number of calories consumed) (12).

NUTRIENT SELECTION BY HUMANS: CARBOHYDRATE CRAVING AND OBESITY

The fact that the nutrient contents (that is, carbohydrates and proteins) of the rat's diet are regulated, and that this regulation involves brain serotonin, led us to inquire whether similar mechanisms might operate in humans, and might shed light on some previously unexplained aspects of human obesity. We were particularly interested in determining whether anecdotal reports that many obese patients suffer from carbohydrate craving were true, and, if so, whether this phenomenon might be reflected in the overconsumption of carbohydrate rich snacks. We also wanted to see whether serotoninergic drugs might suppress such carbohydrate intake in the patients, just as they had been shown to do in normal rats. Finally, we wanted to explore the possibility that the self-reported tendency of obese people to overconsume carbohydrates might represent a kind of "self-medication," that is, that they use foods as though the foods were drugs, to make themselves feel better. (Virtually all of the drugs now used to treat depression share with dietary carbohydrates the ability to enhance serotoninergic neurotransmission; moreover, purely serotoninergic antidepressants like zymelidine and fluoxetine are known to be associated with weight loss and reduced appetite in some depressed people.)

To examine these questions, it was first necessary for us to establish a reliable mechanism for quantifying each subject's eating behavior, particularly for measuring and automatically recording what they ate when they were given access to a full choice of foods and snacks with differing carbohydrate and protein contents. This has been done at the Massachusetts Institute of Technology's Clinical Research Center. Subjects are hospitalized for varying periods and given unlimited access (except at mealtimes) to a vending machine that provides eight or ten different isocaloric foods that are rich in either carbohydrate or protein (14). At each meal subjects are allowed to choose as many portions as they like from among six different foods, also isocaloric and of varying nutrient contents (15).

Our studies have shown the following:

1. Calorie and nutrient consumption *are* surprisingly constant for any individual: Administration of a placebo has no effect on the number (or composition) of snacks chosen per day, and mealtime calorie intake also exhibits little variation (16,17).

2. The great majority of obese people who claim to be carbohydrate cravers very clearly do exhibit such behavior when they are studied in a controlled clinical environment: Many subjects who habitually take three to six carbohydrate snacks per day never eat a protein rich snack at all (15).

3. Their consumption of snacks does not occur at random; rather it is concentrated within one or two periods during each 24 hours, either late in the afternoon, or, more commonly, in the evening (15).

4. The *mealtime* consumption of calories (approximately 1900 in one test group) and of macronutrients (87 g protein, 143 g carbohydrates) tends to be normal, and clearly cannot explain their obesity. However, they also eat, on the average,

700 to 1,000 or more calories per day of virtually pure carbohydrates (i.e., protein free), as snacks.

5. Administration of a "pure" serotoninergic drug, Isomerid
   (D-fenfluramine), selectively suppresses their consumption of
   carbohydrates (14,15): The intake of carbohydrate rich
   snacks declines by about 40% (in subjects receiving 15 mg
   b.i.d. of the drug); mealtime carbohydrate intake declines by
   20% to 25%; mealtime protein intake is not significantly affected. (Too few protein rich snacks are consumed when subjects are receiving placebo to assess whether the treatment
   affects snack protein intake.)

It is also interesting to note the ways that many of the subjects
describe their feelings, before and after they eat carbohydrate rich
snacks. Before the snacks, they use words like "restless, tense, unable to concentrate" to describe themselves; after the snacks they
become "calm, relaxed, able to concentrate," observations compat-
ible with the view that, to some extent, the subjects are *using* the
snacks as a kind of self-medication, to obtain their positive effects
on mood.

To our knowledge, no epidemiologic data are available that
bear on the frequency with which carbohydrate craving occurs as
a major contributing factor in the pathophysiology of obesity.
However, our admittedly uncontrolled experience indicates that
this phenomenon is not at all unusual, and that patients exhibiting it may actually constitute a majority of obese patients, at least
in the region of Boston, Massachusetts. Perhaps their vulnerability
to obesity derives from the fact that serotonin-releasing brain neurons have more than a single function. If *all* that these neurons
did was to participate in feedback loops regulating appetite—if
the neurons were not also involved in the control of mood, and
of such other brain functions as sleepiness, pain sensitivity, and
neuroendocrine secretion—then food intake would not be expected to influence the mood, nor to make some people sleepy,
nor modulate pain sensitivity, nor to affect the release of certain
pituitary hormones. But that is not all that the serotonin-releasing
neurons do: They also are critically involved in certain types of
depression (for example, that seen in the seasonal affective disor-

der syndrome, which also typically is associated with carbohydrate craving (18)). Hence obesity may, in some people, be the unwelcome price for the daily amelioration of mild depression. If this formulation is correct, it may be necessary to use serotoninergic anorexic drugs chronically, just as antidepressant drugs are often so used.

REFERENCES

1. J. D. Fernstrom and R. J. Wurtman, *Sci. Amer.*, **230**, 84 (1974).

2. J. D. Fernstrom and R. J. Wurtman, *Science*, **174**, 1023 (1971).

3. J. D. Fernstrom and R. J. Wurtman, *Science*, 178, 414 (1972).

4. R. J. Wurtman, "Precursor Control of Transmitter Synthesis," in R. J. Wurtman, J. H. Growdon, and A. Barveau, Eds., *Uses of Choline and Lecithin in Neurologic and Psychiatric Diseases*, Vol. V, *Nutrition and the Brain* (R. J. and J. J. Wurtman, Eds., Raven Press, New York, 1979, pp. 1–12.

5. R. J. Wurtman, F. Hefti, and E. Melamed, *Pharmacol. Rev.*, **32**, 315 (1980).

6. J. J. Wurtman and R. J. Wurtman, *Science*, **198**, 1178 (1977).

7. J. J. Wurtman and R. J. Wurtman, *Life Science*, **24**, 895 (1979).

8. R. J. Wurtman, F. Larin, S. Mostafapour, and J. D. Fernstrom, *Science*, **185**, 183 (1974).

9. J. D. Fernstrom and R. J. Wurtman, *Metabolism*, **21**, 337 (1972).

10. J. D. Fernstrom, R. J. Wurtman, B. Hammarstrom-Wiklun, W. M. Rand, H. N. Munro, and C. S. Davidson, *Am. J. Clin. Nutr.*, **32**, 1912 (1979).

11. W. M. Pardridge, "Regulation of Amino Acid Availability to the Brain," in R. J. Wurtman and J. J. Wurtman, Eds., *Nutrition and the Brain*, Vol. I, Raven Press, New York, 1977, pp. 141–203.

12. J. J. Wurtman, P. L. Moses, and R. J. Wurtman, *J. Nutr.*, **113**, 70 (1983).

13. P. L. Moses and R. J. Wurtman, *Life Sciences*, **35**, 1297 (1984).

14. J. J. Wurtman, R. J. Wurtman, J. H. Growdon, P. Henry, A. Lipscomb, and S. H. Zeisel, *Int. J. of Eating Disorders*, **1**, 2 (1981).

15. J. J. Wurtman, R. J. Wurtman, S. Mark, R. Tsay, W. Gilbert, and J. Growdon, *Int. J. Eating Disorders*, **4**, 89 (1985).

16. J. J. Wurtman and R. J. Wurtman, "Impaired Control of Appetite for Carbohydrates in Some Patients with Eating Disorders: Its Treatment with Pharmacologic Agents," in K. Pirke and D. Ploog, Eds., *The Psychobiology of Anorexia Nervosa*, Springer-Verlag, Berlin, pp. 12–21.

17. J. J. Wurtman and R. J. Wurtman, *Int. J. Obesity*, **8**, Suppl. 1, pp. 79–84 (1984).

18. N. E. Rosenthal, D. A. Sack, J. C. Gillin, A. J. Lewy, F. K. Goodwin, Y. Davenport, P. S. Mueller, D. A. Newsome, and T. A. Wehr, *Arch. Gen. Psychiat.*, **41**, 72 (1984).

3

The Satiating Effect of Cholecystokinin

GERARD P. SMITH, M.D.,
and JAMES GIBBS, M.D.
Department of Psychiatry, Cornell University Medical College, and the Eating
Disorders Institute, New York Hospital-Cornell Medical Center, Westchester
Division, White Plains, New York

On the basis of work in rats, we hypothesized that cholecystokinin
released from the small intestine during the ingestion of a meal
acted in a negative feedback manner to terminate that meal (1).
Since then, the hypothesis has been tested extensively. In this
chapter we shall review the relevant results in animal and human
subjects and discuss the therapeutic potential of cholecystokinin
for human eating disorders.

ANIMAL STUDIES

Specificity

The inhibitory effect of cholecystokinin (CCK) on meal size has
been replicated in rats and extended to mice, chickens, pigs,
sheep, and monkeys (2). The inhibitory effect is dose related and
does not show a significant degree of tolerance (3).

The inhibitory effect on food intake is relatively specific in that
equivalent doses have less effect on water intake (1,4). In addition

We are supported by Research Scientist Award MH-00149 (G. P. S.), Research Scientist Development Award MH70874 (J. G.), and Research Grants MH40010, MH15455, and
AM33248. We thank Mrs. Marion Jacobson and Mrs. Jane Magnetti for typing this manuscript.

35

to this behavioral specificity, there is a marked structural specificity (4). The tyrosine residue in the seventh position of the C-terminal octapeptide must be sulfated for the inhibitory effect to occur. This is characteristic of other visceral actions of cholecystokinin, such as stimulation of pancreatic enzyme secretion and contraction of smooth muscle of the gallbladder.

Receptor Sites

Peripherally administered cholecystokinin inhibits eating by acting at a site that is outside the blood–brain barrier because CCK penetrates the blood–brain barrier poorly (5). The current candidate sites in the rat include the pyloric sphincter (6), vagal afferent terminals in the abdomen (7), and the area postrema (8). All of these binding sites discriminate between the sulfated form of CCK-8 and the desulfated form.

Vagal Afferents and Central Processing

The satiating effect of low doses of CCK-8 can be abolished by peripheral abdominal vagotomy (9). The critical vagal lesion involves the afferent fibers (9). Hence, the current mechanism of action appears to be activation of pyloric or vagal receptors by CCK-8. These receptors then produce a propagated action potential up the afferent vagal fibers to the first central synapse in the nucleus tractus solitarus. The subsequent processing of this CCK-induced afferent signal by the central nervous system is not known, but the hindbrain contains sufficient neural complexity to convert the afferent signal into a behavioral decision to stop eating because CCK inhibits food intake in chronic decerebrate rats (10). On the other hand, the paraventricular nucleus of the hypothalamus also appears to be a nodal site for the central processing of the information provided by peripheral CCK because bilateral paraventricular nucleus lesions abolished the satiating effect of peripherally administered cholecystokinin (11).

The Role of Endogenous CCK

In contrast to the reasonably consistent evidence that exogenously administered CCK-8 has a satiating effect, there is no compelling evidence that *endogenous* CCK-8 has a similar effect. For example, when endogenous CCK-8 was released by the administration of trypsin inhibitor, meal size did not change (12). When rats were treated with a specific CCK antagonist before a meal, meal size did not change (13,14). If endogenous CCK had been involved in the termination of eating, the antagonist should have produced an increase in meal size due to the delay in the termination of eating. The only positive evidence concerning endogenous CCK has been two reports suggesting that endogenous CCK released by an oral preload has a satiating effect on a subsequent meal (14,15). This has not been confirmed (16).

Thus, the results on animal studies can be summarized as giving strong evidence for the inhibitory effect of exogenous CCK-8 on food intake, but no clear evidence for the hypothesized role of endogenous CCK-8 in the termination of a meal.

HUMAN STUDIES

There have been six studies of the effect of CCK on eating in humans (17,18). Cholecystokinin inhibits the size of a test meal in lean and obese humans, the effect is dose related, and the inhibition of food intake cannot be explained by the slight symptoms that occur in a minority of the subjects (17). In addition to this effect on meal size, CCK has also been shown to decrease the hunger elicited by the smell, sounds, and sight of food that was being prepared in the room with the subject (19).

Stacher (18) believes that the doses of exogenous CCK required to inhibit food intake in the human may be within the range of plasma CCK that occurs during the ingestion of a meal and, hence, the effect of exogenous CCK in the human may represent a physiological effect of the hormone. This conclusion is inferential and requires more direct testing before it can be accepted.

One of the interesting aspects of the inhibitory effect of CCK on meal size in the human is that subjects do not perceive that they have eaten less or that they are less satisfied by the test meal. Furthermore, in one study, subjects did not snack more often in the afternoon after a smaller meal induced by CCK and they did not advance the time of their evening meal (20). If such observations can be replicated in a larger group of subjects, this would support the evidence that CCK is a novel anorectic agent with unusually specific properties.

Satiety or Sickness

The ability of CCK to decrease food intake in some people without producing any detectable side effects by questionnaire, interview, or videotape is the best evidence that CCK can inhibit food intake without producing malaise or some other form of subtle sickness (17). It would appear to be the crucial evidence in the controversy that arose from animal studies showing that CCK produced a conditioned taste aversion under certain experimental conditions, but not others (21).

Vagal Mechanism

The mechanism of CCK action appears to be similar in the human to that in the rat because vagotomized humans failed to respond to exogenous CCK-8 (22). More work, of course, will be required to establish the vagal mechanism in humans.

THERAPEUTIC POTENTIAL

Despite the encouraging results with CCK in test meal situations, there are significant obstacles to its therapeutic use. These include the inactivity of orally administered CCK, no evidence concerning the safety of CCK when administered chronically, very little evidence about the ability of CCK to inhibit the intake of preferred foods, and the lack of evidence concerning the efficacy of CCK to produce weight loss in humans. When the last two problems have been modeled in the laboratory, CCK has proven effective:

1. Cholecystokinin retained its inhibitory potency against very concentrated sucrose solutions (23).
2. When CCK was administered before each meal in genetically obese rats (24) or in rats with dietary induced obesity (25) for a three week period, CCK produced significant weight loss.

These results suggest that the obstacles enumerated above may not be insuperable, but only further human experiments will give us the answer.

The animal and human studies provide converging support for the ability of exogenous CCK to decrease meal size without producing significant side effects. With this established, current work is focused on two major issues:

1. to determine the details of the vagally mediated action of CCK at its peripheral receptor site and within the vagal projection fields in the hindbrain; and
2. to demonstrate the efficacy and safety of CCK treatment for weight loss in humans.

The results of this work will decide the fate of the CCK hypothesis.

REFERENCES

1. J. Gibbs, R. C. Young, and G. P. Smith, *J. Comp. Physiol. Psychol.*, **84**, 488–495 (1973).
2. J. Gibbs and G. P. Smith, "The Neuroendocrinology of Postprandial Satiety," in L. Martini and W. F. Ganong, Eds., *Frontiers in Neuroendocrinology*, Raven Press, New York, 1984, pp. 223.
3. D. B. West, D. Fey, and S. C. Woods, *Am. J. Physiol.*, **246**, R776 (1984).
4. G. P. Smith, "Gut Hormone Hypothesis of Postprandial Satiety," in A. J. Stunkard and E. Stellar, Eds., *Eating and its Disorders*, Raven Press, New York, 1984, p. 67.
5. W. H. Oldendorf, *Peptides*, 2 (Suppl. 2), 109 (1981).

6. G. T. Smith, T. H. Moran, J. T. Coyle, J. J. Kuhar, T. L. O'Donohue, and P. R. McHugh, *Am. J. Physiol.*, **246**, R127 (1984).

7. T. H. Moran, G. P. Smith, A. M. Hostetler, and P. R. McHugh, *Appetite*, **7**, 282 (1986).

8. T. H. Moran, P. H. Robinson, M. S. Goldrich, and P. R. McHugh, *Brain Res.*, **362**, 175 (1986).

9. G. P. Smith and J. Gibbs, "The Satiety Effect of Cholecystokinin: Recent Progress and Current Problems," in J. J. Vanderhaeghen and J. N. Crawley, Eds., *Neuronal Cholecystokinin*, Vol. 448, N. Y. Acad. Sci., New York, 1985, p. 417.

10. H. J. Grill, D. Ganster, and G. P. Smith, *Soc. Neurosci. Abstr.*, **9**, 900 (1983).

11. J. N. Crawley and J. Z. Kiss, *Peptides*, **6**, 927 (1985).

12. D. Greenberg, G. P. Smith, J. Gibbs, J. D. Falasco, R. A. Liddle, and J. A. Williams, *Soc. Neurosci. Abstr.*, **11**, 557 (1985).

13. S. M. Collins, P. Forsyth, and H. Weingarten, *Life Sci.*, **32**, 2223 (1983).

14. G. Shillabeer and J. S. Davison, *Regul. Peptides*, **8**, 171 (1984).

15. G. Shillabeer and J. S. Davison, "Increased Food Intake in the Rat Caused by Proglumide, the Cholecystokinin Antagonist," in J. J. Vanderhaeghen and J. N. Crawley, Eds., *Neuronal Cholecystokinin*, Vol. 448, N. Y. Acad. Sci., New York, 1985, p. 648.

16. L. H. Schneider, J. Gibbs, and G. P. Smith, *Peptides*, **7**, 135 (1986).

17. G. P. Smith and J. Gibbs, "The Effect of Gut Peptides on Hunger, Satiety, and Food Intake in Humans," in R. J. Wurtman and J. Wurtman, Eds., *Human Obesity*, N. Y. Acad. Sci., New York, 1987, in press.

18. G. Stacher, *Psychoneuroendocrinology*, **11**, 38 (1986).

19. G. Stacher, H. Bauer, and H. Steinringer, *Physiol. Behav.*, **23**, 325 (1979).

20. H. R. Kissileff, F. X. Pi-Sunyer, J. Thornton, and G. P. Smith, *Am. J. Clin. Nutr.*, **34**, 154 (1981).

21. G. P. Smith, J. Gibbs, and P. J. Kulkosky, "Relationships Between Brain-Gut Peptides and Neurons in the Control of Food Intake," in B. G. Hoebel and D. Novin, Eds., *The Neural Basis of Feeding and Reward*, Haer Institute for Electrophysical Research, Brunswick, Maine, 1982, p. 149.

22. M. J. Shaw, J. J. Hughes, J. E. Morley, A. S. Levine, S. E. Silvers, and R. B. Schaffer, "Cholecystokinin Octapeptide Action on Gastric Emptying and Food Intake in Normal and Vagotomized Man," in J. J. Vanderhaeghen and J. N. Crawley, Eds., *Neuronal Cholecystokinin*, Vol. 448, N. Y. Acad. Sci., New York, 1985, p. 640.

23. G. P. Smith and J. Bernz, *Regul. Peptides*, Suppl. 2, S59 (1983).

24. R. G. Campbell and G. P. Smith, *Soc. Neurosci. Abstr.*, **9**, 901 (1983).

25. G. P. Smith and R. G. Campbell, *Appetite*, **7**, 299 (1986).

4

Psychological Factors in the Control of Appetite

C. PETER HERMAN, Ph.D.,
and JANET POLIVY, Ph.D
Department of Psychology, University of Toronto, Toronto, Ontario, Canada

Psychological factors that affect eating include stress, the palatability and salience of food, social influence, and cognitive calculations. It is fruitful to consider these influences as operating by affecting eating either indirectly, by increasing or decreasing hunger or satiety, or directly, independent of the individual's state of deprivation or repletion. We propose a simple model that suggests when hunger or satiety influences may predominate in the control of eating, and when other factors, essentially extrinsic to normal physiological controls on eating, may be expected to manifest themselves. We shall also consider obese vs. normal and dieter vs. nondieter differences in the sorts of factors that govern eating.

Chapters 2 and 3 have addressed the role of various chemicals in the control of appetite. Neurotransmitters and peptides, we are told, are both responsive to what we have eaten and responsible for what we eat, or at least how much we eat. One is tempted or even encouraged to conclude that once we fully understand how our internal chemical messengers operate, the mysteries of why we eat and why we stop eating will have been solved.

One unfortunate by-product of this unfolding success story is that it seems to preempt any possible contribution of psychology to our understanding of why we eat and stop eating. Perhaps

Preparation of this chapter was supported by grants from the Natural Sciences and Engineering Research Council of Canada.

neuropsychologists and physiological psychologists will help explain how chemical messages are transmitted, received, and converted into behavior. But the rest of psychology—what one might call "psychological psychology"—is left without any clear role in this scientific success story.

What about psychological factors in the control of appetite? What psychological factors have been identified? Indeed, are there any worthy of even a bit part in the pageant of appetite regulation?

Perhaps we should start by attempting to indicate what we mean by a psychological factor. Hunger and satiety are psychological, in a way; certainly, we are all familiar with them as feelings or motive states. But although hunger and satiety, as we shall see, are both affected by psychological factors, they themselves have been appropriated by physiological analysts, who think of them mainly as physiological conditions. So if we are to identify *psychological* influences on appetite, we must look for psychological factors that affect hunger and satiety, or perhaps psychological factors that influence eating without affecting hunger and satiety.

According to some physiologically minded researchers, a psychological factor can operate only by influencing hunger or satiety, and not by independently affecting eating. In their view, hunger is defined as what makes us eat, and satiety is defined as what makes us stop; so, by definition, hunger and satiety directly and exhaustively control appetite. Any psychological factor that makes us eat, then, is necessarily mediated by hunger; and any psychological factor that makes us stop eating is necessarily mediated by satiety. The task of the psychologist, at best, is to indicate how a particular psychological factor—such as stress or social pressure—gets converted into the physiological condition of hunger or satiety, which in turn determines eating.

Perhaps this task of reducing psychological factors to their physiological consequences is the best work that we can find. Let us examine some psychological influences on appetite and see how far we have come in understanding how they affect hunger and satiety and ultimately, eating.

As far as we know, there is no definitive list of psychological influences on appetite. Indeed, anyone who would survey the field is faced with the daunting task of organizing a welter of incoherent studies. As a first step, we propose the following categories of major influences, into which most of the variables that have been investigated may be placed: stress, the palatability of the available food, social influence pressures, the perceptual salience of the available food, and, finally, various cognitive considerations governing eating. Let us examine these categories in order.

STRESS

The effect of stress is usually to reduce appetite. People lose their appetites when they are made fearful (1,2), and one of the classic symptoms of depression is loss of appetite (3,4). The suppressive effect of stress on appetite is thought to depend on the psychosomatic fact that stress activates the sympathetic branch of the autonomic nervous system; this activation, in turn, releases stored sugar into the bloodstream, which acts to suppress hunger. Thus, stress reduces appetite by reducing the physiological state of hunger; in other words, the psychological factor of stress directly affects one's physiology, which in turn controls one's appetite. Indeed, close examination of (1) indicates that the suppressive effect of stress on appetite obtains only when experimental subjects are somewhat hungry to begin with. If subjects are not initially hungry, then stress cannot act to reduce their hunger, so it should not suppress their eating relative to that of nonstressed nonhungry subjects. The fact that stress reduces appetite only in subjects who are hungry lends strong support, then, to the notion that stress operates through hunger. Thus, the alleged psychological factor of stress may be thought of at most as an indirect influence on eating. This conclusion reinforces the confidence of the physiological reductionist.

One complication with the foregoing analysis of the effect of stress on eating, however, is that it does not seem to work very well with overweight subjects or dieters. In fact, more often than not (1,2,5–8), such subjects eat more when under stress than when calm. This suggests that maybe in these subjects, stress does not affect eating by way of the mediating influence of hunger; perhaps its influence is more directly psychological. Before we adopt this nonreductionistic psychological explanation, though, we must consider whether it is possible that stress somehow paradoxically increases hunger for such subjects, since if stress somehow increases hunger for some people, then these people will eat more when stressed, and may well end up fat and eager to lose weight (9). Our view—which does not assume as an axiom that hunger and satiety are always involved in the initiation and termination of eating—is that stress does not paradoxically increase hunger for such subjects; rather, stress operates through an entirely different mechanism, unrelated to physiological hunger or satiety. Stress, instead of augmenting hunger, releases the fat person or dieter from the normal cognitive inhibitors that constrain eating. The fat person or dieter does not eat when stressed because of hunger, but rather because the cognitive controls that normally *oppose* hunger are lifted by stress. Dietary vows are abandoned (10).

In summary, stress appears to affect normal weight, nondieting individuals by affecting hunger; it is a classic example of psychosomatic influence. For overweight people and other dieters, however, the effect of stress does not appear to be mediated physiologically. Note that we are not claiming that stress has no physiological representation in the overweight or dieting person; nor do we claim that interference with one's cognitive inhibitions occurs without activity in the neuronal substrate of thought. But for all intents and purposes, the effect is purely psychological, in the sense that hunger and satiety are not centrally involved.

This analysis suggests that defining hunger as what makes you eat and satiety as what makes you stop is not entirely appropriate. We must avoid begging the question, and ask instead, "Do people start eating for reasons other than hunger (or the mere absence of satiety)? And do people stop eating for reasons other than satiety (or the mere absence of hunger)?" As we have seen in the case of stress, we are willing to concede a strong role to hunger in accounting for the effect of stress on normal nondieters; but when it comes to dieters, the classic physiological mediators of hunger and satiety are inadequate to the explanatory task.

PALATABILITY

Probably the single strongest influence on eating is the palatability of the food involved. The observation that palatability increases eating is somewhat tautological, of course, since the palatability of food is determined at least partially on the basis of our willingness to eat a lot of it. Nevertheless, the taste of food has a big impact on our eating, and we may regard taste as a psychological aspect of food. For one thing, it is a perceptual property of food; and moreover, we know that palatability is affected by culture as well as by biology (11).

Before we grant a purely psychological role to palatability, however, we must consider whether it may exert its effect indirectly, like stress, by inducing hunger. Does mouth-watering food make us more hungry? It has been argued (12) that salivation is a good index of hunger, so perhaps foods that make us salivate are in fact making us hungry. This interesting possibility, however, is not quite correct. Salivation is enhanced when one is hungry and encounters a palatable food; but the stimulating effects of hunger and palatability on salivation are not interchangeable. The effect of differential palatability on salivation is strong—maybe even stronger—in subjects who are already very hungry; it is unlikely that these subjects can be made much more hungry by the sight of palatable food. And increasing hunger will not overcome the inhibitory effects of unpalatable food on salivation (see (13) for a discussion). In short, palatability does not create hunger so much as capitalize on it.

Another possibility is that palatability increases eating by decreasing satiety. On the surface, this possibility seems remote, since satiety ought to be responsive to the caloric value of the food, or perhaps to its nutrient content, neither of which is directly or necessarily tied to palatability. You should get just as full eating your most preferred flavor of ice cream as eating your least preferred flavor. Barbara Rolls and her colleagues (14), however, have demonstrated that satiety is decreased when we switch from one food to another; moreover, the ability of a novel food to stimulate more eating compared to a food that one has just been eating is matched by corresponding changes in palatability (15). Thus, it seems that variety may increase palatability, which in turn eliminates satiety, which in turn increases eating. The only problem with this analysis is that Rolls talks about satiety in a special way— as *sensory specific* satiety, or satiety for particular tastes. Her effects appear immediately, rather than after the sort of delay that physiological feedback from the gut would require; and they dissipate just about when physiological satiety should be at its height. In short, increasing palatability may decrease sensory satiety, but it probably does not affect physiological satiety—in which case, palatability's effect on eating is more psychological than physiological.

The proposal that there may be more than one sort of satiety is naturally somewhat disconcerting, but we must recognize that there is probably more than one sort of mechanism that inhibits eating. At the very least, it appears that we may be forced to distinguish between satiety as a physiological feedback signal, indicating that the gut is full or that nutritional needs have been met, and satiety as a sense of having had enough of a particular food, which may be more a matter of perception, novelty, and palatability. The "physiological" sort of satiety is important for regulation of total intake, and perhaps of calories, while the "sensory" sort of satiety is important in ensuring that the organism maintains variety in the diet.

SOCIAL INFLUENCE

There is ample evidence that people are powerfully influenced by the behavior of others, and that this influence extends to eating. Thus, trained confederates instructed to eat either a lot or a little can induce greater or lesser eating in experimental subjects (16,17). It is not inconceivable that seeing others eat a lot might somehow render one physiologically hungry, but in the absence of supporting evidence, we prefer the more common sense assumption that socially induced eating is not dependent on hunger or satiety. Again, we must confront the fact that not all eating occurs in response to physiological pressure. Social pressure affects all sorts of behaviors, and to some extent eating is a social behavior as much as a biological one. We are all familiar with the widespread cultural practice of offering food to guests, irrespective of whether those guests have just eaten. And these guests are expected to eat, whether they are hungry or not; and they do eat, in order not to offend their hosts, who have been so generous with their hospitality. We can attest from personal experience that people who refuse to eat when food is offered socially are regarded as somehow abnormal. Pointing out that one has recently had a complete meal does not excuse one from one's social obligations.

There are many other examples of social influences on eating that operate on a separate track from hunger and satiety. Just as sated people may be induced to eat by an insistent hostess, so hungry people can be induced to forgo available food if the social situation demands it. Women eat less when with a man than when with another woman, in what has been called the Scarlett O'Hara effect (18); Scarlett was taught to eat like a bird when with men, so as to project a more feminine image. And we have shown repeatedly that self-consciousness—the knowledge that another person is aware of how much you are eating—will have a generally suppressive effect, especially for dieters (19).

PERCEPTUAL SALIENCE

The mere visual salience of available food affects one's likelihood of eating it. Food is more likely to get eaten when it is prominently displayed than when it is less salient in one's visual field. Clearly, this effect is mostly attentional, and thus qualifies as an example of a psychological influence on eating. In one study conducted in a fairly upscale French restaurant in Toronto, we (20) had the waitress take dessert orders while holding an attractive piece of cake or pie in one hand, or while empty-handed. She made no comment about the desserts, but merely made them visually available. Diners—especially fat diners—were much more likely to order the displayed dessert than other desserts.

Although the salience of food is an important perceptual influence on eating, we regard it as a relatively weak one compared to other influences. Of course, you can make it a strong influence by using an extreme comparison, such as literally spotlighting the food in one condition and blindfolding the subjects in the control condition. But under normal circumstances, the effect of salience is easily washed out by other considerations. In one recent study in our laboratory (21), normal subjects who were hungry did not eat more of the highly salient food than of the less salient food; they ate a great deal in both cases, suggesting that true hunger may overwhelm the influence of salience. But when comparable subjects were given something to eat beforehand, so that they were not particularly hungry when exposed to the more or less salient food, then the subjects exposed to the salient food ate significantly more than those exposed to the less salient food. In short, if there is no strong biological pressure operating on the subject, and no strong social pressure acting to encourage or constrain eating, then salience effects may emerge. It is of interest to note that in this study, the dieters who had already eaten were not responsive to the salience manipulation. They all ate a great deal, irrespective of salience. For most of them, the initial eating had broken their diets and set them off on a mini-binge. And a bingeing dieter appears to pay little heed to subtleties such as the perceptual salience of the available food, assuming again that even in the less salient case the food is somewhat visible.

Consideration of salience effects reminds us that sometimes psychological factors operate by way of hunger or satiety, as is the case with stress applied to normal eaters, and sometimes psychological factors operate independently of hunger and satiety, as is the case with most social pressures. But to say that a psychological factor operates independently of hunger and satiety should not be taken to mean that hunger and satiety are irrelevant. Rather, hunger and satiety may provide the boundaries within which psychological factors are free to operate (22). If hunger or satiety pressures are strong, the independently operating psychological factors may be overwhelmed. The starving guest may not wait for the other guests to be served before he starts to eat. Yet there appears to be a fairly wide range in which hunger and satiety pressures are fairly weak; and in that range, we may encounter a variety of powerful psychological effects. The interesting question thus becomes, In the normal flow of our daily lives, to what extent is our eating constrained by hunger and satiety, and to what extent are psychological factors free to manifest themselves?

COGNITIVE CONSIDERATIONS

Our research interest in dieters makes us acutely aware of the often predominant role of cognitions in the determination of eating. Indeed, the dieter might almost be defined as one who decides to eat on the basis of something other than hunger and satiety signals. For the most part, she eats—or tries to—in conformity with a set of prescriptive diet rules, which are overlaid on top of (and often obliterate) normal physiological regulation. These rules, concerning how many calories worth of what types of foods are permissible, are devised without much attention to the individual's biological needs. Indeed, dieting might almost be defined as the deliberate defiance of hunger and satiety in the pursuit of a culturally mandated physique. As might be expected, adherence to such cognitively mediated rules renders the dieter's eating patterns incongruent with what we would expect of a normal organism governed mainly by hunger and satiety.

Normal people tend to show compensation to a preload. That is, if you force them to eat varying amounts at Time 1, they will eat compensatory amounts at Time 2, shortly thereafter, so that the total amount eaten, including Time 1 and Time 2, is roughly equal. This sort of compensation is far from perfect, and there is evidence that even in normal eaters there is a strong cognitive component, such that people compensate at Time 2 for what they *think* they ate at Time 1, rather than for what they actually ate (23). Dieters, however, show what we call "counterregulation," eating more at Time 2 after a large load at Time 1 than after a small load at Time 1. This effect is dependent on the dieter's belief that she has blown her diet at Time 1, which somehow justifies her overeating at Time 2. When we give her a pudding at Time 1 and tell her it is high calorie, she acts as if her diet is blown; but the same pudding, described as low calorie, does not constitute a threat to the diet, so the dieter eats a small, diet preserving amount at Time

2 (24). Likewise, a preload of 600 calories of cake suffices to break dieters' diets, whereas 600 calories of salad does not (25).

It appears sometimes that preoccupation with rules and cognitive calculations absorbs dieters to the exclusion of all other potential influences. Indeed, we believe that dieters in many respects allow cognitive considerations to take precedence over all else—including true hunger—in the control of eating. The dieter—self-absorbed and dedicated to achieving a cultural ideal in defiance of her own biology—is a creature unlike any laboratory animal. She reminds us, along with her sisters—those patients with anorexia nervosa and bulimia—that there is more to eating and not eating than hunger and satiety. The psychological influences on eating have not yet even been catalogued; perhaps it is this taxonomic incoherence that leads us all too often to overlook them. But if we are to account for the vagaries of appetite, we must appreciate the frequent and powerful impact of cognitive, social, and perceptual influences on behavior.

REFERENCES

1. S. Schachter, R. Goldman, and A. Gordon, *J. Pers. Soc. Psychol.*, **10**, 91 (1968).

2. R. McKenna, *J. Pers. Soc. Psychol.*, **33**, 311 (1972).

3. A. T. Beck, C. H. Ward, M. Mendelson, J. E. Mack, and J. Erbaugh, *Arch. Gen. Psychiat.*, **4**, 561 (1961).

4. W. W. K. Zung, *Arch. Gen. Psychiat.*, **12**, 63 (1965).

5. C. P. Herman and J. Polivy, *J. Abn. Psychol.*, **84**, 666 (1975).

6. J. Polivy and C. P. Herman, *J. Abn. Psychol.*, **85**, 338 (1976).

7. R. O. Frost, G. A. Goolkasian, R. J. Ely, and F. A. Blanchard, *Behav. Res. Ther.*, **20**, 113 (1982).

8. A. J. Ruderman, *J. Abn. Psychol.*, **94**, 78 (1985).

9. H. Bruch, *Eating Disorders: Obesity, Anorexia Nervosa and the Person Within*, Basic Books, New York, 1973.

10. C. P. Herman and J. Polivy, "Restrained Eating," in A. J. Stunkard, Ed., *Obesity*, Saunders, Philadelphia, 1980.

11. P. Rozin, "Human Food Selection: The Interaction of Biology, Culture, and Individual Experience," in L. M. Barker, Ed., *The Psychobiology of Human Food Selection*, AVI, Westport, CT, 1982.

12. S. C. Wooley and O. W. Wooley, *Psychosom. Med.*, **35**, 136 (1973).

13. O. W. Wooley and S. C. Wooley, *Appetite*, **2**, 331 (1981).

14. B. J. Rolls, E. T. Rolls, and E. A. Rowe, (1982) "The Influence of Variety on Human Food Selection and Intake," in L. M. Barker, Ed., *The Psychobiology of Human Food Selection*, AVI, Westport, CT, 1982.

15. P. Pliner, J. Polivy, C. P. Herman, and I. Zakalusny, *Appetite*, **1**, 203 (1980).

16. R. E. Nisbett and M. D. Storms, "Cognitive and Social Determinants of Food Intake," in H. London and R. E. Nisbett, Eds., *Thought and Feeling: Cognitive Alteration of Feeling States*, Aldine, Chicago, 1974.

17. J. Polivy, C. P. Herman, J. C. Younger, and B. Erskine, *J. Pers.*, **47**, 100 (1979).

18. S. Chaiken and P. Pliner, Women, But Not Men, Are What They Eat: The Effect of Meal Size and Gender on Perceived Femininity and Masculinity. Unpublished manuscript, Vanderbilt University, 1985.

19. J. Polivy, C. P. Herman, R. Hackett, and I. Kuleshnyk, The Effects of Self-attention and Public Attention on Eating in Restrained and Unrestrained Subjects, *J. Pers. Soc. Psychol.*, in press.

20. C. P. Herman, M. P. Olmsted, and J. Polivy, *J. Pers. Soc. Psychol.*, **45**, 926 (1983).

21. J. T. McGree, Physiological and Nonphysiological Influences on Eating: A Test of the Boundary Model. Unpublished M.A. thesis, University of Toronto, 1985.

22. C. P. Herman and J. Polivy, "A Boundary Model for the Regulation of Eating," in A. J. Stunkard and E. Stellar, Eds., *Eating and its Disorders*, Raven, New York, 1984.

23. S. C. Wooley, *Psychosom. Med.*, **34**, 62 (1972).

24. J. Polivy, *Addict. Behav.*, **1**, 237 (1976).

25. J. Polivy, C. P. Herman, and I. Kuleshnyk, More on the Effects of Perceived Preload Calories on Dieters and Nondieters: Salad as a "Magical" Food, University of Toronto, manuscript submitted for publication, 1985.

5

The Role of Food Perceptions in Food Use

MAGDALENA KRONDL, Ph.D.,
and PATRICIA COLEMAN, M.S.
Department of Nutritional Sciences, Faculty of Medicine, University of Toronto, Toronto, Ontario, Canada

Food selection implies choices from a set of available options. We select one food in preference to another, or to accompany another food. Also, we restrict our selection by rejecting specific foods. Thus, nutrient intake and hence food energy intake generated from the ingested macronutrients reflect food use, the outcome of the food selection process. The consequences of food choices in terms of nutrients have received considerable attention, resulting in various nutritional recommendations and dietary guidelines; however, it has become apparent that an understanding of the whole food selection process is critical to the implementation of these recommendations, since this understanding is basic to the prediction and possible modification of eating behaviors.

The purpose of this chapter is threefold. First, we shall explore the food selection/appetite association in terms of the influence of variety on appetite and the sensory role in the acceptance or rejection phenomenon. Next we shall discuss food perceptions as the result of processing of information stored in memory and the contribution of a single food perception/use paradigm to food selection studies. Finally we shall consider the limits on food selection imposed by food-to-food compatibility.

FOOD SELECTION AND APPETITE

The relationship between food selection and appetite is obvious when we accept that food selection determines the degree of variety in the diet. The enhancing effect of food variety on a person's desire to eat has been documented by Rolls and colleagues (1) in experiments in which sandwiches offered with a variety of fillings as opposed to one type of filling resulted in the subjects' eating increased amounts. Their findings were in agreement with those of Schutz and Pilgrim (2) and Siegel and Pilgrim (3). In contrast, the long-lasting negative effect of food monotony on food palatability was documented by Rolls and de Waal (4) even under such drastic conditions as those in refugee camps. According to Köster (5) monotonous and prolonged stimulation not only causes sensory adaptation, but also results in habituation, that is, in a loss of interest in the information presented. New information always attracts our attention and we respond to it, but if the stimulation continues and loses its informational value, we lose interest and may even stop responding to it completely.

THE SENSORY ROLE IN FOOD SELECTION

In food selection, the sensory quality and responses to it are important. The sensory quality is responsible for palatability of foods. Le Magnen (6) defined food palatability as "the contribution of the cephalic sensory activity of the food to the stimulation to eat and to satiation, after some amount of the food has been eaten." Each particular food item possesses its sensory specific satiating power.

Although the role of foods as carriers of nutrients is recognized and nutrient intake assessment is adequately developed, less is known about sensory characteristics and their role in food selection. The sensory quality of food products—their color, taste, odor, and texture—is due to many different components. Flavor-containing substances include nucleotides, amino acids, organic acids, and sugars. They are present in varying amounts in different foods. For example, the flavor of carrots is attributable mainly to amino acids and organic acids (7). Most flavor components and volatile odorous substances are not related to nutritive properties. The flavor is an identifier of a particular family of food products, and of each particular food item, when permanently associated with it. Such a specific and permanent association of taste, smell, and color allows the discrimination and identification of food groups, such as fruits or meats, as well as of particular fruit, such as an apple. The permanent association is essential in food selection, because the "conditioning" of regulatory preference and aversions requires the sensory labeling and therefore the identification of the food (6). Consequently, the sensory properties of foods have important informational value useful in food selection (8). In this manner exposure to ingesta with distinct sensory properties influences the later selection of ingesta with those same sensory properties (9), as in the preference for foods that previously corrected states of deprivation (10). Booth (11) makes the distinction between oral and postingestive consequences of ingestion, and he observes that both kinds of events can serve as unconditional stimuli to reinforce taste preferences.

The experience of pleasantness or unpleasantness, the commonality of the hedonic findings, has led to the idea of a biological basis for certain fundamental taste preferences. From ontogenic studies, starting with the newborn, both animal and human, it appears that there are certain innate determinants of the responses to taste. We have direct evidence of liking or disliking of a particular tastant from photographed facial expressions of the rat (12) and the human infant (13). Innate preferences for sweet foods, such as ripe fruits, have evident survival value for the omnivore in that they often provide a safe and quick source of energy (14). Similarly, innate aversion to bitter tastes (13) may also owe its existence to the selective advantage enjoyed by animals that spontaneously rejected the bitter alkaloids (often poisonous) which are widely distributed in the plant kingdom. Bitter is mostly aversive; sugars are mostly preferred. Saltiness and sourness may be pleasant at low levels (15). Hedonic responses to food stimuli appear to be brainstem reflexes. On top of these are rostral brain structures that add greater complexity to the consumatory behavior of the organism (16). An understanding of the consumatory behavior is the challenge inherent in the study of food selection.

TASTE SENSITIVITY AND HEDONIC RESPONSE TO FOODS

Rozin and Fallon (17) proposed that most food selection behavior in humans is primarily determined by experience. As a direct consequence the recognition of foods could not be prespecified genetically. Nevertheless the importance of studying the genetic component in food selection became apparent after the finding of evidence of heritability in physiological mechanisms affecting food intake (18) and in phenylthiocarbamide (PTC) sensitivity (19,20).

Taste sensitivity, preference, and use of 24 foods were studied on 13 monozygotic and ten dizygotic adult, female twin pairs of comparable family background. Heritability was demonstrated for PTC sensitivity and was found in both reported preference and reported use for unsweetened grapefruit juice and green beans. In terms of preference, a heritability component was indicated in eight foods (bacon, unsweetened grapefruit juice, unsweetened orange juice, unsweetened apple juice, turnips, strawberries, broccoli, green beans) and for use in three of the 24 foods (unsweetened grapefruit, beer, green beans) (21). Environmental adaptation and learning, unmeasured in this twin study, would appear to exert a stronger influence than the genetic component on food related behavior, in agreement with Rozin and Fallon (17).

The relationship between heritability demonstrated for PTC sensitivity and reported preference in four of the eight foods, mainly vegetables of the Cruciferae family containing PTC related compounds, prompted further research. An example of these compounds is the substance goitrin (1,5-vinyl-2-thioxagolidone), which has the same H-N-C=S grouping as and is thought to be responsible for the bitter taste of PTC (19). The design of the study (22) included measurements of sensitivity to PTC, sensory and hedonic ratings for raw and cooked cabbage samples, and assessment of use of cruciferous vegetables for 68 subjectively healthy Caucasian women subgrouped as premenopausal and postmenopausal PTC tasters and nontasters. Sensitivity to PTC and sucrose was measured using a forced choice staircase procedure adapted after Cornsweet (23). Sensory and hedonic ratings were obtained by quantitative descriptive analysis (24). The PTC sensitivity did not deteriorate with age. Although the PTC tasters, particularly in the younger group, appeared to be more aware of differences in flavor intensity and aroma in the raw and cooked cabbage samples than the nontasters, the effect in terms of taster/nontaster differences did not carry over into hedonic responses. The PTC study (22) did not confirm, but also did not negate, the influence of heredity in the sensory mechanism. Nevertheless, the disappearance of the genetic effect in hedonic response again points to the importance of experience with food. There were two differences between the PTC and the twin study. First, PTC tasting is a less reliable model to test genetic influence than a twin study. Blakeslee and Salmon (25) noted wide intraindividual variation in sensitivity to PTC. Second, in the former study we have assessed hedonic responses to tasting actual foods, whereas in the latter perceived liking was recorded. In this connection it is interesting that Hill and Blundell (26) reported differences between young and older populations in judgments of foods to be significantly smaller when food names are read (as is done when food preferences are assessed) than when actual foods are tested. This implies that subjects' concepts of foods remain stable over time. In contrast, judgments of actual foods show an overall age effect. It can be concluded that different results will be obtained depending on the method of determining food preference and that assessing food use is different from assessing food preference.

Irrespective of the genetic influence affecting PTC sensitivity, certain biological influences due to gender and age are evident. Desor and colleagues (27) reported lower sensitivity of sweetness among 9 to 15 year old boys in comparison to girls. Booth and colleagues (28) have shown that age depresses olfactory and gustatory acuity. In addition, Schiffman (29) demonstrated that with age, there was decreased ability to discriminate between foods that were homogenized and judged blindfolded.

The effect of experience on sensory responses has been re-

ported in a number of studies. For example, Solms (7) demonstrated cultural differences in assessment of both flavor and texture of mango fruit. In contrast to Europeans, who have shown a
wide range in their judgment of the sample's sweetness, most of
the East Africans did not consider this fruit sweet enough; for
most of the West Africans it was too sweet. The judgment of the
texture displayed other differences. Whereas the sample of mango
was not firm enough for the Europeans it was too firm for West
Africans.

Whether genetic, hormonal, or metabolic, the biological traits
that evidently are influencing sensory acuity are not as readily
seen in liking or disliking foods. This phenomenon appears to be
more under environmental influences. Thus the adaptability to
preferring or rejecting foods appears to be a viable mechanism
important even for man in search of his food.

THE CONCEPT OF FOOD PERCEPTIONS

Since the sensory responses not only do not fully explain liking of
foods but even less their selection, other mechanisms must be at
play. Olson (30) and Barker (31) suggest an information processing
approach involving memory to the understanding of food acceptance and emphasize the internal cognitive mechanisms of people
who are engaged in food selection. These reflect the subject's past
experiences represented cognitively as knowledge and they have
an effect on the information processes that occur. These major
processes have been adapted to food selection and are shown in
Figure 5-1. Olson (30) theorizes about the way existing knowledge
can affect the cognitive processes involved in interpreting new information. He suggests that it is useful to think about knowledge
structures as memory schemata. The schemata idea is based on the
perspective that attention, perception (encoding), memory, and
other cognitive processes are highly related, intertwined phenomena. Moreover, it is assumed that the purpose of these processes
is the formation of a meaningful interpretation of the world. If so,
the sensory information available from all senses to a person must
be organized and amended in terms of some coherent framework

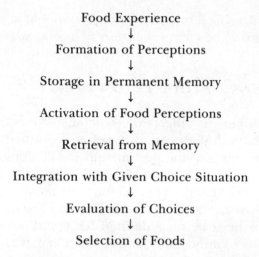

Figure 5-1. Major processes in food selection. (After Olsen 1981.)

or structure. According to Olson, schemata are the large number of structures or frames that allow and facilitate such organization and coherence in our perceptions. Over a lifetime of experience, people form vast numbers of memory schemata. Each schema consists of the content of acquired knowledge as well as the organizing structure or framework for interrelating that content; schemata are interrelated among themselves as well. Olson emphasizes that it is important to recognize that schemata or knowledge structures are highly context specific. Another important characteristic of schemata-knowledge structures is that well-developed, frequently used schemata may appear to operate automatically, without any conscious awareness of their operations. Such well-learned schemata allow the rapid judgments and evaluations typical of our everyday life.

On previous encounters with the food, the subject encodes the food, that is, assigns meaning to it in the form of a symbolic code, or a category of meaning to the incoming sensations received from a sense receptor. Incoming sensations from the sense receptor and existing knowledge structures held in memory must interact for the encoding or comprehension to take place. This analysis points out the central, critical role of the perception that is held in memory in explaining the comprehension of a food attribute.

MEASUREMENT OF FOOD PERCEPTIONS

Food use by a person reflects the outcome of a relationship between the food and the person. It depends on the nature of the food item, the status of the person, and the circumstances of the particular eating context. According to Booth (32) it is a dynamic process that may change from moment to moment. The assessment of food use cannot be static in design or interpretation. The measurements must be on a defined food, with a person whose temporary state of mind, body, and environment is also controlled and monitored for all relevant aspects. Booth suggests that despite the complexity of the inputs to momentary use, it may be possible to find a unity on the output side and "the disposition of an individual to use a particular food or drink in particular circumstances at a moment in time might be a viable unit of behavior and attitude." He is of the opinion that we might proceed on the basis that search, approach, and consumption have a motivational unity, except to the extent proved otherwise. Booth (32) further suggests that "people's perceptions and intentions can be evident in their words. Appropriate questions posed in a properly monitored context should elicit symbolic answers, which reflect the same motivational organization as determines their spontaneous intake." The questioning must avoid biasing the respondent. Booth indicates that a behavioral disposition is fundamentally the same as an attitude, except that the latter can be expressed in words or some other symbolic response. Verbal statements are difficult to verify; nevertheless, objective behavioral measurements are biased because of environmental constraints.

We have explored one approach to the study of the perceived determinants of food use with implications for sensory evaluation, food product development, or nutrition intervention. This approach evaluates people's attitude to foods in terms of motives or reasons for dietary choice. Four of the profiles are motives determining use or nonuse: satiety, tolerance, taste, and healthfulness.

The other profiles of reason are more condition-specific: price, prestige, and convenience.

In designing methodology to assess the role of food perceptions in food selection, the perceptions were defined as the encoding of food experiences according to

a. external and internal realities,

b. the messages of the stimuli that are conveyed by the nervous system to the integrative centers where thinking and evaluation take place, and

c. the resultant interpretation of the messages with feedback from past experiences (33).

The strength of various perceived attributes of selected foods was assessed with Likert-type scales (34). Simultaneously frequency of use of these foods was measured and correlated with the food perceptions.

THE SIGNIFICANCE OF PERCEPTIONS OF FOODS IN FOOD USE

Food experiences or practices are affected by social factors, availability, and accessibility of foods. Food has to be an available commodity on the market. This is the condition for a choice. In addition, foods have to be accessible. The accessibility of food is governed by the available food dollar, as well as by the time and skills of the consumer and the facilities that can be utilized for storage and food preparation. Social factors are superimposed on existing food-related values stemming from the individual's particular cultural heritage. Food advertising and nutrition education may be included along with social factors; the former influences social value of a food and the latter leads to the imposition of specific health attributes on food (35). Before the social factors affect a person's food selection, they are individually evaluated in terms of relevance to the act of selecting a specific food. Below, we shall consider how food accessibility and perception of its social components affect food use, the outcome of food selection.

The societal definition of price is the quantity of one thing that is demanded in exchange for another. When income level approaches the poverty line, and the balancing of the total budget for the needs of housing, clothing, transportation, and food is in question, price consideration may limit the range of foods used. Foods perceived to be too expensive for the budget will be eliminated and the foods selected will be mainly those required for the satisfaction of hunger and maintenance of life. Thus foods such as bread, flour, potatoes, sugar, and jams, which are viewed as staple items, hold a static position regardless of income and price fluctuations. Significant consumption increases were observed in the United Kingdom for dairy, meat, fish, fruit, and vegetable products when income increased. A reversed trend was demonstrated for condensed milk and margarine (36).

The perception of the price of food differs from the societal concept. It is the cost of food in relation to personal wants and needs. Reaburn and colleagues (37) used a five point scale with wording indicating price, ranging from "very cheap" to "very expensive" in measuring the perception of price. The perception of price relates to a number of influences other than dollar value for unit quantity. These investigators identified such factors as quantities of food needed to satisfy family appetite, and rejection or waste of food such as broccoli by children, as affecting the perception of price of that particular food. In addition, the form in which the food is purchased and the cost of other ingredients used in combination with the food before serving also relate to the perception of price. In considering the effect of price perception on food use, it could be assumed that frequency of use of a specific food would fluctuate with its market cost. It was therefore postulated that if a food is perceived as being low priced it would be associated with higher consumption. Conversely, if an item is perceived to be high priced, it would be associated with low consumption. Nevertheless, the study by Reaburn and colleagues (37) indicated a more complicated situation. It included 112 low income urban homemakers who had to balance rising prices against low incomes. Only one food (pork or in children, liver) out of 52 foods studied showed a significant negative correlation with price perception. This suggests that frequency of use of a particular food

may decrease with increased food price perceptions among eco-
nomically and socially deprived persons but only for a very small
subset of foods included in the study.

Convenience of foods generally is defined as anything that saves
or simplifies work and adds to one's ease or comfort. More specifically, convenience foods are those that have services added to the
basic ingredients to reduce the amount of preparation required
in the home (38). By using this definition as a standard, all foods
including raw, semiprocessed, or completely processed items can
be rated on an appropriate scale. Reaburn and colleagues (37) described the two extremes of convenience as "takes very long and
is difficult to prepare," and "very quick and easy to prepare."

Convenience-oriented consumption has been identified by Anderson (39) as representing a focal point between rising affluence
and the increasing significance of time. On this basis it could be
hypothesized that people with real or perceived time constraints
would be more frequently inclined to choose foods perceived as
highly convenient. Convenience as a food choice motive fluctuates
in importance depending on age, sex, income, and education of
the food "gatekeeper," as well as with location, rural or urban, of
the household (40). Most North Americans under 30 years of age
readily accept convenience foods, presumably because they were
regularly exposed to them early in their lives. In their study, Reaburn and colleagues (37) found that convenience was not a significant food choice motive among low income housewives. Obviously
other factors, such as eating qualities, may be more relevant. In a
study of the elderly (22), living alone was found negatively to affect
the use of Brassica vegetables. This type of vegetable requires
preparation and it was used less by persons living alone presumably because of inconvenience. Perceived convenience seems to
be important only in the selection of specific foods by specific
population groups.

Prestige of foods is some measure of the position of the food in
a hierarchy relative to society's values. It is a difficult term to define and uniform criteria for the evaluation of prestige do not
exist. Peer influence, as an external social cue, may induce changes
in values and affect the rationale for assigning status value to
foods. Reaburn and colleagues (37) have assessed food prestige as

the appropriateness of the food for guests or for special occasions. It was interesting to note that even within a list of common and inexpensive foods, different prestige values were represented. For example, the low prestige value of beef liver was constantly indicated. Such fresh foods as juice, strawberries, homemade bread, and homogenized milk were considered higher in prestige than the frozen and preprocessed types. Nevertheless only two out of 52 foods were found to have prestige significantly associated with use.

From the preceding evidence, it is apparent that the perceptions of price, convenience, and prestige in the social category play a minor role in influencing the use of foods and do not fully elucidate the mechanism of food selection. Perceived healthfulness and the sensory perceptions were included in two other studies, one of 194 elderly people, and another of 135 adolescents. In both studies, the perception and use of eight selected foods were compared (41,42). The sensory factors included taste, satiety, and tolerance of foods. The scales used for measuring perceptions in these studies are described elsewhere (41–43).

Among both populations, irrespective of age and gender, taste was the factor most often associated with use of foods. Unpleasant tastes, such as those associated in the young with beef liver, fish, or squash, seemed to lead to food rejection. This finding was in agreement with others (17,44). Although older people are labeled as having decreased taste acuity (28), they may rely on memory in their perception of taste. It has been suggested that with adequate instructions, there may be no deficit in the ability to use imagery as a semantic factor in elderly people (45). Perceived healthfulness ranked second to taste for elderly people but fourth for adolescents as an associative factor to food use on the basis of the strengths of the simple correlations. Adolescents may correctly assess the healthful qualities of foods but do not apply this information to food use. As Becker (46) states: "according to the health belief model, when individuals do not believe they are susceptible to becoming ill, and their actions will not bring serious consequences, action will not occur." Since the adolescents in the study all considered themselves to be healthy, this may explain why the perception of healthfulness of foods ranked lower than taste, satiety, and tolerance in terms of motives for food use. Perceptions of satiety and tolerance ranked second and third as factors of signifi- cance in relation to use of selected foods among the young people. One could assume that for the young, who are in the anabolic stage of life, the association of satiety with food as well as postin- gestional feelings will be much more pronounced than among el- derly people. The elderly are at another stage of life, when they are attempting to maintain health, and thus healthfulness of foods has greater value for them than for the young person (Figure 5– 2).

In the studies of food perceptions, age and gender effects were observed. The age-related effects on the perceptions were much more numerous than the gender-related effects, suggesting that accumulated experience plays an important role in the creation of perceptions and that with age, people become more diverse in their link with food (47). Where gender effects occurred, the con- tribution to the total variance in food use was low. Females, partic-

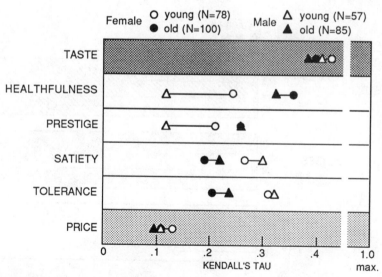

Figure 5–2. Correlations between food use and food perceptions for young and elderly people for eight foods—whole wheat bread, beef liver, frozen fresh fillet, 2% milk, margarine, lettuce, squash, apple juice.

ularly teenagers, because of their desire for thinness, seemed to place a higher value on healthfulness of foods than the males (Figure 5-2). The prestige or social connotation of foods also appeared to be more important to females than to males.

An interesting finding suggesting the effect of experience on food use was observed for two vegetables, lettuce and squash, among the elderly people (Figure 5-3). Correlations between food use and perceptions of taste and healthfulness among both males and females, and tolerance among males, were stronger in the case of the squash than the lettuce. Because of the high degree of technological input necessary for production and storage, lettuce in Canada has increased in availability since World War II. In contrast the squash, cheap to grow and to store, was readily available in prewar rural families and hence was probably more familiar in the youth of today's seniors. According to Kuo (48), early exposure is important for later food selection. Also Capretta (9) and Rozin (14) suggested that exposure to ingesta with distinct sensory properties influences the later selection of ingesta with those same sen-

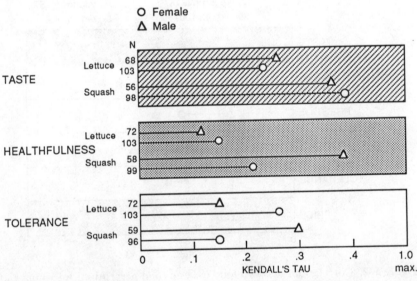

Figure 5-3. Correlations between food use and food perceptions of two vegetables by elderly men and women.

sory properties. The time and length of exposure to these two vegetables suggest an explanation for the difference in perception
and use between them.

In studies of both adolescents and elderly people, not all of the
variance of food use was explained by food perceptions. It is recognized that in an area as complex as food behavior, many interrelated factors are operating and consideration of food combinations, meal patterning, and food substitutions would be necessary
to explain fully the remaining variance.

CHANGEABILITY OF FOOD PERCEPTIONS

Capretta's (9) principle of stimulus relevance, implying that the
act of consumption must be related to the consequences of consumption in order to modify food preference, confirms Rzoska's
(49) rat experiment and Rozin's (14) observations. Just as physical
traits, such as specific receptors for sweet or bitter, were subject to
natural selection, the same process has occurred with behaviors in
that some behavioral patterns that appear intelligent in fact arise
from phylogenetic memory rather than from learning. In rats and
humans an important group of behavioral strategies in feeding
belong to this category.

First there is the approach to new foodstuffs. On one hand, food
sampling is essential in adjusting to new situations and maintaining intake from a wide variety of food sources but, on the other,
any potential new food could be poisonous. Thus omnivores exhibit ambivalent behavior towards new foods. They are both hesi-
tant and curious. Wild rats approach a new food with great cau-
tion, taste it, and then wait some time before consuming any more
(49). This strategy increases their chances of identifying poisonous
foods without killing themselves in the process of doing so; however once a new food has been tasted and does no harm, it becomes a safe familiar food and is no longer approached hesitantly
(14).

A study of dietary acculturation of Chinese adolescent immigrants to Canada has documented a similar behavioral pattern
(48). Interestingly, as will be shown later, the perception of foods

has changed simultaneously with frequency of use within two generations. The study involved an immigrant population that consisted of 36 first generation and 18 second generation Chinese adolescent males, age 14 to 16 years. Subjects born in the orient, mainly Hong Kong, were included in the first generation group, those born in Canada or the United States, with both parents born in the orient, were considered as second generation. The mean length of residence in Canada for the first generation group was 7.2 years. An age and sex matched Canadian adolescent group (N = 44) was included in the study for comparison. This group was selected to include only those whose parents and both grandparents were of British descent.

Acculturation changes of the Chinese groups were assessed mainly by a comparison of perceptions and food use of the two generation subgroups. It was assumed that the acculturation process would be reflected in the changes occurring between the first and second generation, and that food perceptions of the second generation boys would approach those of their Canadian peers. The generation comparison was validated with a language use acculturation index (51).

Measurements of flavor ratings reflected a stronger liking for desserts, snacks, fast foods, and common beverages by second generation Chinese than by first generation. A similar strong hedonic liking of these foods was reported by the Canadian adolescent sample. Thus taste profiles of the second generation Chinese boys approached those of the Canadians; however, the higher number of foods rated as very good by the Canadian boys suggests that acculturation of flavor perception is not complete by the second generation.

According to Moskowitz and colleagues (52) cultural differences in flavor preferences may be mere reflections of habitual diets. One would predict the increased "liking" of foods to be paralleled by their higher use. This was in fact the case, since many of the well-liked foods were used more frequently by the more acculturated second generation Chinese boys (51).

Generation differences in the perceived health values of foods suggested a higher familiarity with "Western" nutrition concepts with acculturation. A greater knowledge of nutrition was also exhibited by the Canadian boys. The more neutral health ratings given to foods by the first generation Chinese boys than by the second generation Chinese or Canadian boys may relate to the differences in health belief systems of the two cultures. In the oriental hot-cold humoral balance of health concepts, emphasis is placed on culturally defined hot and cold properties of foods, food combinations, and their contribution to specific physiological states (53). Within this belief system, health values of individual items taken out of context of actual consumption may be more ambiguous and therefore considered neutral. In contrast, in the Western culture, where emphasis is placed on the nutrient content of food, the distinction between nutrient rich and poor foods is reinforced through the school system and the media. It is therefore not surprising that these principles are reflected in the perceived healthfulness of foods by the Canadian and the more acculturated second generation Chinese boys. The food use patterns (50), however, suggest that the acquired nutrition knowledge was not put into practice by the second generation Chinese boys. Food items given more negative health ratings were not necessarily consumed less frequently by the second generation Chinese boys.

Foods typically used in the company of friends were considered more prestigeous by the second generation than by the first generation Chinese adolescents. In contrast, little acculturation in terms of prestige was found for foods usually eaten at home with one's family. The prestige construct, which measured the degree to which foods were appropriate to be eaten with friends, may not have been relevant for the latter food group. A number of foods, such as doughnuts or honey-buns, chips, and French fries, were also eaten more frequently by the second generation Chinese boys than by their less acculturated peers, indicating that the perceived prestige influenced their use (50).

Although the use of only a small percentage (15%) of all food items assessed changed with acculturation, these can be considered markers of a general trend towards the higher use of highly processed foods and lower food variety within the vegetable food group. The use of several of the highly processed foods by the second generation Chinese boys tended to be similar to that of the

Canadian boys. This may be a consequence of the similarly high pleasure and prestige values given to such foods by these two groups. In contrast the lower use of many of the vegetable items observed in the second generation Chinese did not parallel a similar low use by the Canadian boys. Thus acculturation of use of many foods cannot be predicted simply on the basis of food habits of the predominant culture. It seems that use patterns of foods with high prestige and pleasure values are the most readily adaptable.

Furthermore, many more food use differences were found between the Chinese and Canadian boys (53%), than between the two Chinese subgroups (15%), indicating that acculturation of food use patterns was not nearly complete by the second generation.

In agreement with Jerome (54), several patterns of dietary acculturation were observed. In general, the wider range of food use frequencies in the first generation subgroup reflects a process of experimentation with new and traditional foods. Following this phase, foods are either incorporated as core foods or rejected from the diets of the more acculturated second generation subgroup. Alternatively, some items become more sharply defined as peripheral or marginal foods. Most of the dietary changes found, in parallel to the observations of Caster (55), involved peripheral and marginal foods. New foods were typically introduced at this usage frequency. As well, peripheral and marginal foods were more readily abandoned. The core diet was more resistant to change.

The strength of associations between perceptions and frequency of use of 48 foods suggests that the acculturation of the family, as reflected in the availability of foods, strongly influenced food use. The highest correlation was found between these two variables. Familiarity, or the length of time since a food was first tried, was also an important determinant of use, as was taste acceptability. In contrast, the prestige and healthfulness perceptions, those which are most clearly manipulated by peer and school influences, were only weakly correlated with use. This indicated that peer pressure and nutrition education have little direct impact on the food habit acculturation process.

Interactions between the food perceptions for Chinese boys were examined (Table 5-1). A strong association was found between home availability and taste acceptance, indicating that foods available frequently at home were perceived as tastier. Availability at home was also strongly related to food familiarity, which in turn enhanced taste acceptance. One interpretation, therefore, may be that foods introduced at an earlier age, mainly through the family, were perceived as tastier and this in turn enhanced their use.

It was interesting that high correlations were also found between prestige and both healthfulness and taste, indicating that these perceptions modify food selection; probably they do so indirectly through a stronger use determinant such as taste. Foods of higher peer value and those that were perceived as healthier were also considered tasty and therefore used more often. Furthermore, foods perceived as good for one's health were considered more prestigeous by this group. These relationships suggest that the school system does have some impact on food practices; however it is much weaker than that of the family. Furthermore, taste acceptance seems to be an important vehicle through which the weaker food selection motives can act.

Interestingly when only treat foods, or foods that the boys bought for their own use, were looked at separately, an almost identical set of interrelationships was found. Home availability, reflecting the family influence, was the strongest determinant of use. However, because the Kendall Tau correlations do not neces-

Table 5-1. Intrarelationships[a] Between Food Perceptions and Food Use of Chinese Boys (n = 54).

	Prestige	Healthfulness	Taste	Familiarity	Availability
Availability	0.147	0.173	0.226	0.325	1.00
Familiarity	0.220	0.148	0.233	1.00	
Taste	0.323	0.206	1.00		
Healthfulness	0.206	1.00			
Prestige	1.00				

[a]Median Kendall Tau associations based on 46 foods.

sarily imply causality, it is also possible that the availability of foods at home is to some extent dependent on the adolescent, who may introduce certain foods to the family if he finds them acceptable (50). On immigration, adaptation to the diet of the host country resembles the process of assimilation by the young of the diet prevailing in society. The adaptation of elderly people to the products of the new food technologies follows a similar pattern. The change occurring in food patterns will depend on the strength of established perceptions and desire and opportunity to assimulate and accept the change.

FOOD-TO-FOOD COMPATIBILITY

Research in the area of human food selection has been limited with few exceptions to studies of single food items. Since most foods are eaten in combinations with other foods as mixed dishes or as a meal, acceptance of individual foods can be altered by combining with other foods. Since food preferences and food use are mostly environmentally dependent and culturally transmitted, as shown in previous sections, food combinations are likely to be under strong cultural influence. A study (56) was designed in which four foods termed "central" foods and 40 combinant foods were presented to experimental subjects with instructions that the combinant foods were to be positioned on a circular grid containing one of the central foods at its center. This was repeated with each central food. The distance between a central food and each combinant food indicated the degree of compatibility. The data were processed so that the compatibility of each combinant food with each central food was established for three cultural groups, Chinese, European, and West Indian. The numbers of women representing these cultures were 18, 10, and 11, respectively. In spite of the small subject sample size and the restricted list of foods, there was a strong indication that a protein food is most apt to be selected as the core of food patterns and that vegetables contribute most to the variability in food combinations. These results may have been limited because of the imposed restriction in the option of foods or the influence of past emphasis on the nutritional significance of protein in the diet. Interestingly, women of European and Chinese origin appeared to have more rigid rules for what is an appropriate food combination than women of West Indian origin (Table 5-2). This study offers yet another explanation for a part of the variation in human food selection and confirms the important role of culture, a factor implying food memory.

Food selection mechanisms are both physiological and behavioral. Unfortunately the complexity of the processes and the biological as well as experiential uniqueness of each individual (57) have led to the division and oversimplification of the separate mechanisms. Only recently is there a base of knowledge sufficient to allow suggestions that the quantitative and qualitative aspect of eating along with the individuality of people and the uniqueness of specific foods are all part of an integrated system. Decisions whether to consume a particular food have been known to be made mostly on an individual intuitive and largely subconscious basis. The arguments presented in this chapter, based on data mostly from our findings, confirm this statement. More specifically they document further that food likes are learned and little influenced by genetic endowment. In addition, they confirm that sensory attributes of foods are generally the most important in food selection but are complemented by other motives, depending mostly on the person's age but less on gender. Changes in food selection that occur gradually are accompanied by changing perceptions of food, mainly of hedonic food meanings. Limits to food selection are identified as cultural food compatibility. These could be due to memory schemata. Food selection is closely related to perceived taste, depending on the palatability of food, which in turn affects food intake. Since food intake has been related to a desire to eat (58), loosely termed appetite (11), we may conclude that food perceptions, usually considered psychological factors, contribute to the control of appetite. From our research, perceptions of foods are at the root of food selection. They are connected with specific food experience, with the strongest input from overall sensory response reinforced by other social attributes at different stages of development, well being, and social context.

Food selection is a dynamic adaptive process subject to change,

Table 5–2. Differences in Food Combinations with Four Central Foods[a] among Chinese, European, and West Indian Women[b]

Ethnic Group Favoring Combination	Foods Combined with Central Foods[c]			
	Cola Beverages	French Fries	Chicken	Brussels Sprouts
Chinese	Chinese cabbage	—	Bok choy Choy sum	—
European	Brussels sprouts Tomato	Tomato	Potato Brussels sprouts Cauliflower Endive Green beans	Potato Beef

West Indian			
Bok choy	Cabbage	Beef	Potato
Choy sum	Okra	Pork	Beef
Plantain	Plantain	Cabbage	Bok choy
Okra	Tomato	Okra	Cabbage
	Fruit juice	Plantain	Cauliflower
	Fruit drink	Tomato	Green onions
	Water	Fruit drink	Plantain
		Fruit juice	Snow peas
		Milk	Tomato
		Soft drink	
		Water	
Total differences in food combinations among three ethnic groups	7	7	18	9
% of possible combinations[d]	18	18	46	23

[a] Foods selected as representative of items that determine food patterning among specific ethnic groups.
[b] All groups first generation immigrant women.
[c] Food combinations significantly different ($p \leq .05$) from other two ethnic groups.
[d] Maximum number of possible combinations = 39.

its rate and degree of change dependent on the character and strength of the food stimulus, the sensitivity of the respondent, and the intensity of the experience. It has implications for molding not only the dietary patterns of today but also those of tomorrow.

REFERENCES

1. B. J. Rolls, *Nutrition Bull.*, **5**, 8 (1979).

2. H. E. Schutz and F. J.Pilgrim, *Psychol. Reports*, **4**, 559 (1958).

3. P. S. Siegel and F. J. Pilgrim, *Am. J. Psychol.*, **71**, 756 (1958).

4. E. T. Rolls and A. W. L. de Waal, *Physiol. and Behavior*, **34**, 1017 (1985).

5. E. P. Köster, "Time and Frequency Analysis: A New Approach to the Measurement of Some Less Well-known Aspects of Food Preferences?" in J. Solms and R. L. Hall, Eds., *Criteria of Food Acceptance*, Forster Verlag, Zurich. 1981.

6. J. Le Magnen, "Neurophysiological Basis for Sensory Mediated Food Selection," in *Criteria of Food Acceptance*, J. Solms and R. L. Hall, Eds., Forster Verlag, Zurich, 1981.

7. J. Solms, Genner-Ritxmann. *Lebensmittel Tech.*, **18**, 3 (1985).

8. J. E. Blundell, "Problems and Processes Underlying the Control of Food Selection and Nutrient Intake," in *Nutrition and the Brain*, Vol. 6, R. J. Wurtman and J. J. Wurtman, Eds., New York, Raven Press, 1983, pp. 164–218.

9. P. J. Capretta, "Establishment of Food Preferences by Exposure to Ingestive Stimuli Early in Life," in *Learning Mechanisms in Food Selection*, L. M. Barker, M. R. Best, and M. Domjan, Eds., Baylor U. Press, Texas, 1977, pp. 99–121.

10. L. H. Revusky, *Psychonomic Sci.*, **7**, 109 (1969).

11. D. A. Booth, "Food-conditioned Eating Preferences and Aversions with Interoceptive Elements: Conditioned Appetites and Satieties," in N. S. Braveman and P. Bronstein, Eds., *Experimental Assessment and Clinical Applications of Conditioned Food Aversions.* Ann. N.Y. Acad. Sci. Vol. 443, 1985, pp. 22–41.

12. H. J. Grill, "Introduction: Physiological Mechanisms in Conditioned Taste Aversions," in N. S. Braveman and P. Bronstein, Eds., *Experimental Assessments and Clinical Applications of Conditioned Food Aversions*, Ann. N.Y. Acad. Sci., Vol. 443, 1985, pp. 67–87.

13. J. Steiner, "The Human Gustofacial Response," in J. F. Bosens, Ed., *Fourth Symposium on Oral Sensation and Perception-Development of the Fetus and the Infant*, U.S. Gov. Print Office, Washington, D.C., 1973, pp. 254–278.

14. P. Rozin, "The Selection of Foods by Rats, Humans and Other Animals," in J. Rosenblatt, R. A. Hinde, C. Beer, and E. Shaw, Eds., *Advances in the Study of Behavior*, 6, Academic Press, New York, 1976, pp. 21–76.

15. C. Pfaffmann, *Psychol. Res.*, **42**, 165 (1980).

16. S. W. Kiefer, "Neural Medication of Conditioned Food Aversions," in N. S. Braveman and P. Bronstein, Eds., *Experimental Assessments and Clinical Applications of Conditioned Food Aversions*, Ann. N.Y. Acad. Sci., Vol. 443, 1985, pp. 100–109.

17. P. Rozin and A. E. Fallon, "The Acquisition of Likes and Dislikes for Foods," in J. Solms and R. L. Hall, Eds., *Criteria of Food Acceptance,* Forster Verlag, Zurich, 1981, p. 36.

18. J. Wade, J. Milner, and M. Krondl, *Am. J. Clin. Nutr.,* **34,** 143 (1981).

19. R. Fischer, "Genetics and Gustatory Chemoreception in Man and Other Primates," in M. R. Kare and O. Maller, Eds., *The Chemical Senses and Nutrition,* Johns Hopkins Press, Baltimore, 1967, pp. 61–81.

20. N. G. Martin, *Ann. Hum. Genet.,* **38,** 321 (1975).

21. M. Krondl, P. Coleman, J. Wade, and J. Milner, *Hum. Nutr.: Appl. Nutr.,* **37A,** 189 (1983).

22. M. Krondl, A. Niewind, M. Shrott, and M. Latta, "Influence of Genetic Factors on Food Selection," Abstract, Am. Coll. Nutr., 25 Ann. Meeting, Boston, Massachusetts, 1984.

23. T. N. Cornsweet, *Am J. Psychol.,* **75,** 485 (1962).

24. H. Stone, J. Lidel, S. Oliver, S. Woolsey, and R. C. Singleton, *Food Techn.,* **28,** 24 (1974).

25. A. F. Blakeslee and T. N. Salmon, *Proc. Natl. Acad. Sci.,* **21,** 84 (1935).

26. A. J. Hill and J. E. Blundell, *J. Psychiat. Res.,* **17,** 203 (1982/83).

27. J. A. Desor, O. Maller, and L. S. Greene, "Preference for Sweet in Humans: Infants, Children, and Adults," in J. M. Weiffenbach, Ed., *Taste and Development,* U.S. Dept. of HEW, Bethesda, Maryland, 1977, pp. 161–172.

28. P. Booth, M. B. Kohrs, and S. Kamath, *Nutr. Res.,* **2,** 95 (1982).

29. S. Schiffman, *J. Geront.,* **32,** 586 (1977).

30. J. C. Olson, "The Importance of Cognitive Processes and Existing Knowledge Structures for Understanding Food Acceptance," in J. Solms and R. L. Hall, Eds., *Criteria of Food Acceptance,* Forster Verlag, Zurich, 1981.

31. L. M. Barker, "Building Memories for Foods," in L. M. Barker, Ed., *The Psychobiology of Food Selection,* AVI, Westport, Conn., 1982, pp. 85–100.

32. D. A. Booth, "Momentary Acceptance of Particular Foods and Processes that Change It," in *Criteria for Food Acceptance,* J. Solms and R. L. Hall, Eds., Foster Verlag, Zurich, 1981, pp. 49–68.

33. D. Lau, M. Krondl, and P. Coleman, "Psychological Factors Affecting Food Selection," in J. R. Galler, Ed., *Nutrition and Behavior,* Plenum, New York, 1984, pp. 397–415.

34. M. Krondl and D. Lau, *Can. J. Pub. Health,* **69,** 39 (1978).

35. M. Krondl and D. Lau, "Social Determinants in Food Selection," in L. M. Barker, Ed., *The Psychobiology of Human Food Selection,* AVI, Westport, Connecticut, 1982, pp. 139–152.

36. J. C. McKenzie, "Economic Influences on Food Choices," in M. Turner, Ed., *Nutrition and Lifestyles.* Applied Science Pub., London, 1979.

37. J. Reaburn, M. Krondl, and D. Lau, *J. Am. Dietet. Assn.,* **74,** 637 (1979).

38. M. Glicksman, "Fabricated Foods," in *CRC Critical Reviews in Food Technology,* Vol. 2, Chemical Rubber Co. Press, Cleveland, Ohio, 1971.

39. W. T. Anderson, *J. Market Res.,* 8, 179 (1971).

40. G. L. Tinklin, N. E. Fogg, and L. M. Wakefield, *J. Home Ec.,* **6,** 26 (1972).

41. M. Krondl, D. Lau, M. A. Yurkiw, and P. H. Coleman, *J. Am. Dietet. Assn.,* **80,** 523 (1982).

42. R. S. George and M. Krondl, *Nutr. and Behav.,* **1,** 115 (1983).

43. D. Lau and M. Krondl. "Food Perception—Nutritional Significance in Aging," Abstract. XIII International Congress of Nutrition, Brighton, U.K. 1985.

44. E. Randall and D. Sanjur, *Eco. Food Nutr.,* **11,** 151 (1981).

45. A. M. Fullerton, *J. Geront.*, **38**, 326.

46. M. H. Becker, L. A. Maiman, J. R. Kirscht, D. P. Haefner, and R. H. Drachman, *J. Health and Soc. Behav.*, **18**, 348 (1977).

47. M. L. Axelson and M. P. Penfield, *J. Nutr. Ed.*, **15**, 23 (1983).

48. L. Y. Kuo, *The Dynamics of Behavior Development: An Epigenetic View*, New York, Random House, 1967.

49. J. Rzoska, *Brit. J. Anim. Behav.*, **1**, 128 (1953).

50. N. Hrboticky and M. Krondl, Dietary Acculturation of Chinese Adolescent Immigrants *Nutrition Research* (in press).

51. N. Hrboticky and M. Krondl, *Appetite*, **5**, 117 (1984).

52. H. R. Moskowitz, K. N. Sharma, H. L. Jacobs, S. D. Sharma, and V. Kunraiah, *Sciences*, **190**, 1217 (1975).

53. L. C. Hsu, *Ecol. Food Nutr.*, **3**, 303 (1974).

54. N. W. Jerome, "Diet and Acculturation: The Case of Black-American Migrants," in N. W. Jerome, R. F. Kandel and G. H. Pelto, Eds., *Nutritional Anthropology: Contemporary Approaches to Diet and Culture*, New York, Redgrave, 1980, pp. 275–325.

55. W. O. Caster, *Ecol. Food Nutr.*, **9**, 241 (1980).

56. A. C. Niewind, M. Krondl, and T. Van't Foort, "Combination of Foods in Terms of Food Compatibility, Abstract, XIII International Congress of Nutrition, Brighton, U.K., 1985.

57. R. M. Pangborn, "Individuality in Responses to Sensory Stimuli," in J. Solms and R. L. Hall, Eds., *Criteria of Food Acceptance*, Forster Verlag, Zurich, 1981, pp. 177–219.

58. J. Kennedy, "The Effect of Acetylsalicylic Acid Use and Dose, Osteoarthritis, and Psychosocial Factors on the Appetite and Energy Intake of Free Living Elderly Persons," M.Sc. Thesis, University of Toronto, 1985.

6

Pharmacological Modification of Appetite

ANN C. SULLIVAN, Ph.D.,
CHERYL NAUSS-KAROL, Ph.D.,
SUSAN HOGAN, Ph.D.,
and JOSEPH TRISCARI, Ph.D.
Research Division, Hoffmann-La Roche Inc., Nutley, New Jersey

The pharmacological modification of appetite is the only drug therapy approved at present to treat obesity. Extensive clinical experience has indicated that currently available appetite suppressants are useful as short term supplements to weight reduction programs employing nutritionally sound diets. However, long term use of these anorectic drugs by obese patients is restricted because of side effects, potential addiction liability, and the development of tolerance. These limitations coupled with the recognized need for drugs to treat obesity have encouraged the search for new types of pharmacological agents to decrease food intake. This chapter will review marketed anorectic drugs, including their usefulness and limitations, and research compounds in clinical and preclinical evaluation.

IDEAL ANORECTIC AGENT

It is useful to consider the properties of the ideal anorectic agent as a guide to evaluate future drugs. As outlined in Table 6-1, such an agent should reduce food intake consistently and produce a sustained reduction of body weight through a selective decrease

79

Table 6-1.   Properties of The Ideal Anorectic Agent

- Sustained reduction of food intake producing weight loss through a selective reduction of body fat levels with sparing of body protein.
- Improved compliance with a sound weight reduction program of diet and exercise.
- Prevention of weight regain once ideal body weight has been reached.
- No adverse side effects or abuse potential with chronic administration.

in body fat levels, while sparing body protein. The ideal anorectic agent should accelerate weight loss and prevent its regain once ideal body weight has been reached. In addition, no adverse effects should be seen upon chronic administration, thus providing clear evidence of long term safety. The use of such an agent should also improve the compliance of individuals on a sound weight reduction program consisting of diet and exercise.

Because of the multiple compensatory systems that function to maintain elevated body fat levels in obese patients, several drugs with different mechanisms of action may be required to achieve significant efficacy, particularly in severe forms of obesity.

MARKETED ANORECTIC DRUGS

Table 6-2 lists anorectic drugs currently available in the United States by prescription. Numerous clinical trials have been conducted with these agents and their efficacy in promoting weight reduction is summarized in reviews conducted in 1975 by Scoville (1) and in 1978 by Sullivan and Comai (2). The Scoville review comprised data from over 200 controlled, double-blind studies from a total of 7,725 obese patients treated with the drugs listed in Table 6-2. Since no significant differences in efficacy were observed among all the anorectic drugs, data on drug treated patients were combined and compared to placebo treatment. As shown in Table 6-3, after four weeks of treatment and at the end of treatment (up to 12 weeks) significantly more patients on anorectic drugs than placebo lost weight, although the percent of

Table 6–2. Prescription Anorectic Drugs Currently Available in the United States

Generic Name	Propriety Name	Drug Enforcement Administration Schedule
Amphetamine	Dexedrine, Obetrol	II
Methamphetamine	Desoxyn	II
Phenmetrazine	Preludin	II
Benzphetamine	Didrex	III
Phendimetrazine	Plegine and others	III
Diethylpropion	Tenuate, Tepanil	IV
Fenfluramine	Pondimin	IV
Mazindol	Sanorex, Mazanor	IV
Phenetermine	Fastin and others	IV

patients continuing to lose weight dropped sharply with time. The key finding of these studies was that the use of an anorectic drug will produce a rate of weight loss of 0.5 lb per week greater than that achieved by placebo administration.

In 1978 Sullivan and Comai (2) evaluated the results of a series

Table 6–3. Weight Loss in Patients Treated with Anorectic Drugs[a]

	Placebo	Anorectic
Number of patients	4,543	3,182
Weight loss after 4 week treatment		
% Achieving 1 lb/wk	46	68
% Achieving 3 lb/wk	4	10
Weight loss at end of treatment		
% Achieving 1 lb/wk	26	44
% Achieving 3 lb/wk	1	2

[a]Adapted from (1). Active drugs included: D-Amphetamine, D,L-Amphetamine, Methamphetamine, Phenmetrazine, Benzphetamine, Phendimetrazine, Phentermine, Chlorophentermine, Chlortermine, Mazindol, Diethylpropion, Fenfluramine.

of double-blind clinical studies of over 5,000 obese patients in which anorectic agents were used for two to 60 weeks. Their findings were similar to those reported by Scoville, that is, that anorectic drugs produced an average weight loss of 0.6 lb per week greater than that achieved by placebo. Again, efficacy was similar with all anorectic drugs.

Chronic use of these anorectic drugs is restricted because of the development of tolerance to the appetite suppression, potential addiction liability, and side effects such as nervousness, insomnia, and tachycardia for all but fenfluramine. Since fenfluramine is a central nervous system depressant, its side effects are sedation and some gastrointestinal intolerance. For a detailed summary of the side effects of marketed anorectic drugs see (3). Increased weight gain is often associated with withdrawal of anorectic drugs. Since all anorectic drugs appear to produce comparable efficacy, there is no justification in the use of schedule II (increased risk for abuse potential) anorectic drugs for antiobesity therapy.

The use of certain anorectic drugs in experimental animal studies has helped us identify and understand the multiple physiological mechanisms involved in appetite regulation. Amphetamine, mazindol, and diethylpropion appear to produce their anorectic effects by interacting with the catecholaminergic system (4,5), whereas fenfluramine functions through the serotonergic system (6).

NOVEL ANORECTICS ACTING
THROUGH SEROTONERGIC MECHANISMS

It has been reported that antidepressant therapy, particularly with tricyclic drugs, frequently results in weight gain. However, clinical studies with three antidepressants that are specific serotonin uptake inhibitors, zimelidine, femoxetine, and fluoxetine (for review see (7)), have shown either no weight gain or reduced body weight in certain depressed patients.

Zimelidine was evaluated for antiobesity effects in 18 nondepressed obese female patients receiving zimelidine for eight weeks or placebo for eight weeks in a double-blind crossover study (8).

Zimelidine significantly decreased appetite as measured by subjective hunger ratings and produced a significantly greater weight loss (2.5 kg) than placebo over the eight week treatment period. Although zimelidine produced useful effects, it was withdrawn from the market in 1983 because of severe adverse reactions, which included fever and elevated hepatic enzyme levels in approximately 1.5% of patients (9,10).

Femoxetine was studied in a double-blind placebo controlled trial of 81 obese patients (11). Average weight loss during the 16 week study was 5.3 kg and 1.5 kg for the femoxetine treated and placebo groups, respectively. This degree of weight reduction is similar to that described above for marketed anorectics.

Fluoxetine is undergoing extensive clinical evaluation for both depression and weight control and several reports have appeared in abstract form (12,13). A series of studies were conducted in either depressed patients or nondepressed obese patients and weight loss was observed in both groups. During eight weeks of treatment in a study of 120 depressed patients, fluoxetine treated patients (20–80 mg per day) lost a mean of 4.5 kg, whereas placebo patients lost a mean of 1.4 kg (12). Weight loss was proportional to initial body mass index. In a subsequent eight week study of nondepressed obese patients, the fluoxetine group receiving 60 mg per day lost a mean of 4 kg, compared to a mean loss of 0.6 kg for the placebo group (12). Fluoxetine (mean dose 65 mg) was compared to benzphetamine (mean dose 97 mg) or placebo for eight weeks in a total of 150 nondepressed obese subjects (13). Average weight losses of 10.4, 8.7, and 3.6 lbs were reported for groups receiving fluoxetine, benzphetamine, and placebo, respectively. Safety data from over 3,000 depressed patients treated with fluoxetine at doses of 20–80 mg per day have also been reported in abstract form (14). Nausea, nervousness, drowsiness, tremor, and excessive sweating were reported significantly more frequently with fluoxetine than with placebo treatment.

CHOLECYSTOKININ

Cholecystokinin (CCK) has been evaluated for its potential role as a short term satiety signal (for reviews see (15,16)), in addition to its well-known function as an endogenous peptide stimulating gall bladder contraction and release of digestive enzymes from the pancreas in response to a meal. The initial report of the satiating effects of CCK in rats (17), has stimulated work in several other species (15), including the human (18–21).

Recent clinical studies have employed the synthetic C-terminal octapeptide of cholecystokinin (CCK-8), since this has the full spectrum of biological activity of CCK. An early trial of 14 normal volunteers given CCK-8 (20, 40, or 80 μ/kg) by intravenous (iv) or subcutaneous (sc) injection 10 or 20 minutes prior to a liquid formula test meal did not show any consistent changes in liquid meal intake (18). In addition, two subjects receiving 80 ng/kg iv and one subject receiving 40 ng/kg iv experienced adverse effects of nausea, headache, flushing, diarrhea, and abdominal cramping. No side effects were reported by the 10 subjects receiving 20 ng/kg of CCK-8 by either iv or sc administration.

Three recent clinical trials have examined the effects of CCK-8 by iv infusion on the intake of solid or semisolid meals in lean and obese subjects (19–21). Table 6–4 summarizes the effects of intravenous infusions of CCK-8 to lean (19) and obese (20) subjects on semisolid meal size and duration. Each study was conducted in a randomized, double-blind crossover manner. Significant reductions in both meal size and duration were observed in both lean and obese subjects receiving CCK-8. Five of the 12 lean subjects reported a "sick" sensation during CCK-8 treatment and not during saline treatment, although this was not related to satiety and

Table 6–4.   Effect of Intravenous Infusion of CCK-8 to Lean and Obese Subjects on Meal Size and Duration[a]

Subjects	Treatment	Meal Size g	Meal Duration minutes
Lean	Saline	644	9l4
Lean	CCK-8	522[b]	7.8[b]
Obese	Saline	977	12
Obese	CCK-8	852[b]	9.4[b]

[a]Adapted from (19) and (20); iv infusion of CCK-8 (4 ng/kg/min).
[b]$p < .05$ compared to saline treatment.

the sensation was apparently mild. A higher incidence of a "sick" sensation was also reported by obese subjects during CCK-8 infusion. No other side effects were reported by either lean or obese subjects.

Sixteen healthy volunteers receiving single iv infusions of either saline, 4.6 ng/kg/minute CCK-8, or 9.2 ng/kg/minute CCK-8 were studied for effects on intake of sandwiches (21). Subjects receiving the higher dose of CCK-8 reduced intake by 50% ($p < .01$) and reported less hunger ($p < .02$). Those receiving the lower dose reduced their intake by 17% ($p < .05$) and also reported less hunger ($p < .05$). No side effects were reported.

In summary, the synthetic octapeptide of CCK apparently produces early termination of a meal, since obese and lean subjects ate less as a result of a shorter meal duration. Thus, CCK-8 appears to mimic the satiation inducing effects of CCK reported in rats. These results are encouraging, although CCK-8 has no practical use as an antiobesity agent, since it must be administered parenterally and has a short duration of effect. If an orally active, longer acting analog of CCK could be developed, it would be of significant interest as an appetite suppressant.

OPIOID ANTAGONISTS

The potential importance of opioids in the regulation of appetite and drinking behavior is being explored because synthetic and endogenous opioid agonists such as morphine and β-endorphin, respectively, stimulate both food and water intake. However, the response to opioid agonists is not always uniform and may depend on the class of opioid receptors involved as well as species, strain, or genetic differences.

Naloxone, an opiate antagonist, suppressed food intake in rodents and in both obese and lean humans (22–25). However, naloxone has a short duration of action. As shown in Figure 6-1, food intake was suppressed only during the first hour of a three hour meal in lean rats given 5 mg/kg of naloxone subcutaneously 30 minutes before the meal. In addition, naloxone is not orally active and must be administered parenterally.

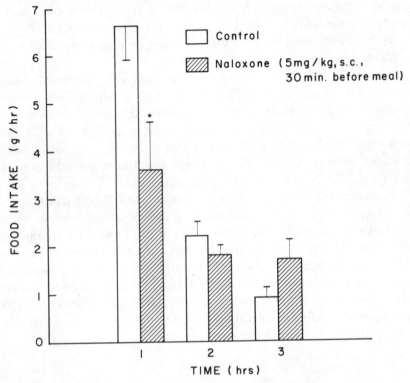

Figure 6-1. Effect of nalaxone (5 mg/kg, sc, 30 minutes before a meal) on food intake of Sprague-Dawley rats trained to consume a 3 hour meal.

Naltrexone is an orally active analog of naloxone, which is a potent, long acting opioid antagonist. In an early study when naltrexone was used as a narcotic antagonist, subjects reported a decrease in appetite during treatment (26). Reduced food intake was also reported by six out of ten opiate free volunteers after naltrexone administration (27). However, subsequent trials in obese patients have not shown significant antiobesity effects (28-30).

Naltrexone at a daily dosage of 50 mg and 100 mg in an eight week outpatient study had no significant effect on body weight of obese male and female subjects when grouped together (28). However, when analyzed by sex, women given naltrexone showed a mean weight loss of 1.7 kg compared to a mean weight gain of 0.1 kg ($p < .05$) by women given placebo. Six of the 54 subjects completing this trial had increases in one or more liver function tests while taking naltrexone. In a subsequent ten week outpatient trial of naltrexone at 200 mg daily in obese men and women, no significant differences in weight loss between patients receiving naltrexone (1.8 kg) and placebo (1.5 kg) were observed and no sex effect was seen (29). Furthermore, liver transaminase levels were elevated to twice baseline values in three of 21 subjects given naltrexone. Finally, in a 28 day, crossover design, inpatient study of obese men receiving daily doses of 100 to 300 mg of naltrexone, no significant effects on food intake or body weight were observed (30).

These negative results of naltrexone on body weight in obese humans could be due to naltrexone's weak activity against kappa receptors (31), the subtype of opioid receptor believed to play a major role in the opioid modulation of feeding behavior (32). Additional studies are needed, particularly involving the effects of opioid antagonists on subtypes of obesity, if these can be defined, such as those characterized by high endogenous β-endorphin levels, stress induced eaters, or bulemics.

CHLOROCITRIC ACID

Chlorocitric acid (Ro 21-7716) is the result of a search for anorectic agents that mimic peripheral signals involved in appetite regulation. Although its precise mechanism of action is unclear, rodent studies demonstrate that chlorocitric acid reduces gastric emptying (Fig. 6-2) and alters the circulatory levels of certain gut hormones (33). Furthermore, chlorocitric acid was shown to act synergistically with CCK-8 in reducing food intake in rats (34).

Food consumption was reduced in a dose dependent manner by the oral administration of chlorocitric acid to lean and obese rats and dogs (35,36). Chronic administration of chlorocitric acid to rats produced a significantly reduced rate of weight gain caused by a selective reduction of body fat levels; protein levels were unchanged. No tolerance developed to the anorexia produced by chlorocitrate and no side effects were observed.

In an 18 day inpatient study the effect of chlorocitrate was investigated in obese men (37). Attractively presented food was avail-

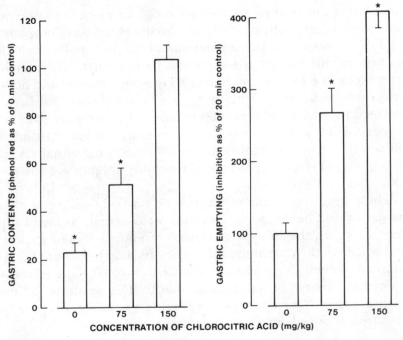

Figure 6-2. Effect of chlorocitric acid on gastric emptying in Sprague-Dawley rats as measured by gastric contents of phenol red (left panel) and inhibition of gastric emptying (right panel). Gastric contents of phenol red were determined 20 minutes after the oral administration of phenol red and compared to the stomach contents of an initial group (0 minute control) in which the animals were killed immediately following intubation with phenol red. Inhibition of gastric emptying was determined by comparing the amount of phenol red left in the stomachs of control and chlorocitric acid treated rats 20 minutes after the oral administration of phenol red, to that of the initial group (0 minute control).

able ad libitum to all subjects and food intake was monitored covertly by using the Platter Service Method (38). Consumption of a single test meal using the Universal Eating Monitor (39) was measured during the placebo and drug treatment periods. After a four day baseline period when placebo capsules were given three times a day, a 14 day treatment phase of the double-blind study was initiated with each subject randomly assigned either chlorocitrate or placebo for the first seven days, followed by alternate treatment for the next seven days. Chlorocitrate was administered one or two hours before each meal at a dose of 300 mg (total daily dose 900 mg). Obese men receiving chlorocitrate gained an average of 1.6 kg less during the seven day treatment period than during the placebo period ($p < .02$). Food intake was reduced by approximately 1,644 kcal during the week of drug treatment, but this difference was not significant. On the average, subjects given chlorocitrate ate less and had a slower initial rate of eating on the Universal Eating Monitor; however these differences did not reach statistical significance. No clinically significant adverse effects were observed. This study, suggesting that chlorocitrate produces an antiobesity effect, needs to be confirmed and extended to longer term clinical trials.

REFERENCES

1. B. A. Scoville, "Review of Amphetamine-Like Drugs by the Food and Drug Administration: Clinical Data and Value Judgments," in G. A. Bray, Ed., *Obesity in Perspective: Proceedings of the Fogarty Conference*, Washington, DC, U.S. Govt. Ptg. Office, 1975.

2. A. C. Sullivan and K. Comai, *Int. J. Obes.*, **2**, 167 (1978).

3. G. A. Bray, "Drug Therapy for the Obese Patient," in L. H. Smith, Jr., Ed., *The Obese Patient*, Philadelphia, W. B. Saunders, 1976.

4. R. Samanin, "Central Mechanisms of Anorectic Drugs," in F. G. de las Heras and S. Vega, Eds., *Medicinal Chemistry Advances*, Pergamon, New York, 1981.

5. S. Dobrzanski and N. S. Doggett, *Psychopharmacol.*, **66**, 297 (1979).

6. J. Duhault, L. Beregi, and R. du Boistesselin, *Curr. Med. Res. Opin.*, **6** (Suppl. 1), 3–14 (1979).

7. L. Lemberger, R. W. Fuller, and R. L. Zerbe, *Clin. Neuropharmacol.*, **8**, 299 (1985).

8. R. J. Simpson, D. J. Lawton, M. H. Watt, and B. Tiplady, *J. Clin. Pharmacol.*, **11**, 96 (1981).

9. C. N. Sawyer, J. Cleary, and R. Gabriel. *Br. Med. J.*, **287**, 1555 (1983).

10. B. S. Nilsson, *Acta. Psychiatr. Scand.* **68** (Suppl. 308), 115 (1983).

11. J. Smedegard Kristensen and P. Christiansen, *Ugeskr. Laeg*, **144**, 938 (1982).

12. L. R. Levine, *Alim. Nutr. Metab.*, **7**, 21 (1986).

13. J. M. Ferguson and J. P. Feighner, *Alim. Nutr. Metab.*, **7**, 19 (1986).

14. R. L. Zerbe, *Alim. Nutr. Metab.*, **7**, 22 (1986).

15. J. Gibbs and G. P. Smith, *Fed. Proc.*, **45**, 1391 (1986).

16. G. Smith, *Int. J. Obes.*, **8** (Suppl. 1), 35 (1984).

17. J. Gibbs, R. C. Young, and G. P. Smith, *J. Comp. Physiol. Psychol.*, **84**, 488 (1973).

18. F. L. Greenway and G. A. Bray, *Life Sci.*, **21**, 769 (1977).

19. H. R. Kissileff, F. X. Pi-Sunyer, J. Thornton, and G. P. Smith, *Am. J. Clin. Nutr.*, **34**, 154 (1981).

20. F. X. Pi-Sunyer, H. R. Kissileff, J. Thornton, and G. P. Smith, *Physiol. Behav.*, **29**, 627 (1982).

21. G. Stacher, H. Steinringer, G. Schmierer, C. Schneider, and S. Winklehner, *Peptides*, **3**, 133 (1982).

22. E. Trenchard and T. Silverstone, *Appetite*, **4**, 43 (1983).

23. R. L. Atkinson, *Clin. Endocrinol. Metab.*, **55**, 196 (1982).

24. E. Trenchard and T. Silverstone, *Int. J. Obes.*, **6**, 217 (1982).

25. M. Kyriakides, T. Silverstone, W. Jeffcoate, and B. Laurance, *Lancet*, **1**, 876 (1980).

26. D. Smith, "Method for Inducing Anorexia," U.S. Patent Application Number 27,270 (1979).

27. L. Hollister, *Drug and Alcohol Dependence*, **8**, 37 (1981).

28. R. L. Atkinson, L. K. Berke, C. R. Drake, M. L. Bibbs, F. L. Williams, and D. L. Kaiser, *Clin. Pharmacol. Ther.*, **38**, 419 (1985).

29. R. Malcolm, P. M. O'Neil, J. D. Sexauer, F. E. Riddle, H. S. Currey, and C. Counts, *Int. J. Obes.*, **9**, 347 (1985).

30. C. A. Maggio, E. Presta, E. F. Bracco, J. R. Vasselli, H. R. Kissileff, D. N. Pfohl, and S. A. Hashim, *Brain Res. Bull.*, **14**, 657 (1985).

31. T. M. Egan and R. A. North, *Science*, **214**, 923 (1981).

32. J. E. Morley and A. S. Levine, *Peptides*, **4**, 797 (1983).

33. J. Triscari, S. R. Bloom, T. Gaginella, T. O'Dorisio, and A. C. Sullivan, *Int. J. Obes.*, **9**, A101 (1985).

34. J. Triscari, S. Hogan, D. Nelson, W. Danho, and A. C. Sullivan, *Fed. Proc.*, **44**, 1162 (1985).

35. A. C. Sullivan, W. Dairman, and J. Triscari, *Pharmac. Biochem. Behav.*, **15**, 303 (1981).

36. J. Triscari and A. C. Sullivan, *Pharmacol. Biochem. Behav.*, **15**, 311 (1981).

37. S. Heshka, C. Nauss-Karol, A. Nyman, K. Reisen, H. R. Kissileff, K. P. Porikos, and J. G. Kral, *Nutr. Behav.*, **2**, 233 (1985).

38. K. P. Porikos, A. C. Sullivan, B. M. McGhee, and T. B. Van Itallie, *Clin. Pharmacol. Ther.*, **27**, 815 (1980).

39. H. R. Kissileff, G. Klingsberg, and T. B. Van Itallie, *Am. J. Physiol.*, **238**, R14 (1980).

7

Regulation of Food Intake During Pregnancy and Lactation

PEDRO ROSSO, M.D.
Department of Pediatrics, Catholic University, Santiago, Chile

Pregnancy and lactation determine an increase in food intake which is limited to the duration of these periods and whose relative magnitude varies in different species. In general, species with large litters increase food intake proportionally more than those with small litters. For example, the rat increases its nonpregnant food consumption 100% during pregnancy and approximately 450% during lactation (1). In contrast, a woman needs to increase food intake only 10% to 15% during pregnancy and 20% to 25% during lactation (2) (Fig. 7-1). It is generally assumed that the greater food consumption of pregnancy and lactation reflects the maternal adaptation to the nutrient drain caused by the fetus and later by milk production. It is, probably, the apparent obviousness of the situation that has discouraged researchers from investigating the mechanisms involved. In fact, the number of studies on this subject is surprisingly low considering that pregnancy and lactation are states of physiological hyperphagia and, as such, they offer the unique possibility of exploring mechanisms of food intake control in the absence of experimental manipulation.

Most of the experimental data on food intake regulation during pregnancy and lactation derive from studies conducted in rats. In this species greater food consumption begins early in pregnancy, reaches a peak during midgestation, and decreases somewhat near term (1). Food intake increases progressively during lactation and near weaning values are usually 2.5 times those observed during

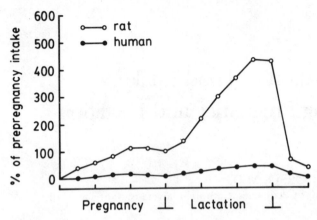

Figure 7-1. Changes in food intake during pregnancy and lactation in humans and rats. Values represent % change over prepregnancy levels. Data on pregnant women adopted from various sources and on pregnant rats from (1).

pregnancy (1). After weaning there is a sudden drop in food intake, which returns to prepregnancy levels. This pattern of changes is similar to that observed in humans, but, as mentioned earlier, proportionally much greater. In this respect, it is important to point out the present scarcity of information regarding food intake during pregnancy and lactation in well-fed healthy women. The available studies have important limitations such as reduced sample size or the possibility that intake was influenced by cultural and economic factors, or both.

APPETITE CONTROL DURING PREGNANCY

Besides changes in food intake, pregnancy also induces changes in food preferences, at least in humans, which seem to be the only mammalian species where the phenomenon has been observed. A study in a middle income American population (3) found that foods frequently craved were ice cream, sweets and candy, fruits, and fish. Aversions focused on red meat, poultry, and certain sauces. The single most important change was a substantial increase in milk consumption, while coffee consumption was drastically reduced. Somewhat similar changes seem to occur in other populations and countries, although in general national and ethnic food habits strongly influence the types of food preferred or avoided (4–6).

The causes of the changes in food preferences are unknown. The most accepted theory is that they reflect a reduction in taste acuity, a phenomenon that has been known for many decades (7), but has never been explored in detail. The change appears to be so subtle that most women are unaware of it; however, unconsciously they begin to prefer more tasty and highly flavored foods. Most likely, other factors participate as well, including common pregnancy "side-effects" such as nausea and heartburn.

Pica, which is craving for nonnutritional substances, is also more common among pregnant women. In the United States the consumption of laundry starch (amylophagia) has been described in low income black women (5,8). Studies have investigated a possible link between this type of pica and the existence of iron deficiency with inconclusive results (9,10).

The mechanisms responsible for the increased appetite of pregnancy remain unknown. Comparisons between changes in maternal food intake and fetal growth suggest that nutrient drain by the fetus has little, if any, influence on maternal appetite. As shown in Figure 7–2, maternal food intake begins to increase shortly after week 12 of gestation, when fetal body mass is too small to determine significant nutrient demands. Later on, between weeks 20 and 40 of gestation, daily caloric intake begins to fall off while fetal body weight and, presumably, nutrient requirements are increasing linearly. Similarly, maternal metabolic rate, reflected by oxygen consumption, increases linearly throughout gestation (12). Thus, the pattern of change seems unrelated to the changes in maternal food consumption.

Little is known about maternal physical activity during the course of pregnancy, except that it declines during the second half. Since daily physical activity is an important determinant of caloric needs, it seems logical to attribute to a reduced physical activity the decline in maternal food intake observed at this stage.

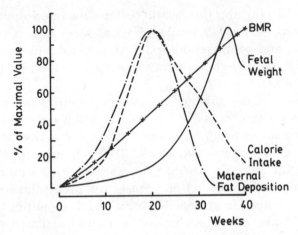

Figure 7-2. Changes in maternal calorie intake, maternal fat deposition, fetal weight, and basal metabolic rate (BMR) during pregnancy. Values are expressed as % of maximal change. Data on calorie intake adopted from (11). Maternal fat deposition, BMR, and fetal weight adopted from (13).

The estimated pattern of maternal fat deposition during gestation closely resembles that of maternal food consumption (14). The most obvious explanation is a causal relationship between these two variables. Early in gestation, when maternal food intake is greater than fetal needs, the extra calories are deposited as fat. Later on, when maternal caloric intake decreases and fetal needs are greater, the rate of fat deposition decreases proportionally.

As a whole, the data mentioned above suggest that factors other than fetal and maternal metabolic needs are influencing the increase in appetite. Landau has proposed that progesterone could be such a factor (15).

Progesterone is secreted in large quantities by the placenta. Plasma levels of this hormone increase throughout pregnancy, reaching near term concentrations considerably higher than those observed in the luteal phase of the menstrual cycle (16). Plasma levels of estrogen, which antagonizes the effect of progesterone in various target tissues, also increase during gestation (16).

The gestational increase of progesterone occurs earlier than that of estrogen. For this reason the first half of gestation is considered to be under the influence of progesterone while during the second half estrogen would neutralize some of the effects. Both hormones have been linked to the changes in appetite observed during the menstrual cycle. A double-blind study conducted in a group of nutrition students found that daily caloric intake was 10% to 20% below average during the postmenstrual days, when progesterone levels are lowest (17).

In the virgin rat progesterone administration determines an increase in food intake and changes in body composition similar to those of pregnancy, namely fluid retention and fat deposition (18). In female baboons progesterone given during the midpoint of the menstrual cycle also leads to an increased food intake (19). These data have been interpreted as an indication that progesterone is an appetite stimulant, but an alternative explanation is that estrogen is an appetite depressant. Either effect could be direct or mediated by another substance or metabolite influenced by these hormones. Landau hypothesizes that the appetite increase elicited by progesterone is secondary to changes induced in amino acid metabolism (15). This author believes that progesterone increases amino acid catabolism in liver and by way of this effect reduces plasma free amino acid concentration which, in turn, would be the signal triggering the change in appetite. Studies by Landau have shown that progesterone administration increases net protein catabolism in both female and male subjects fed a constant diet (20). However, the observation that despite its metabolic effect progesterone fails to influence appetite in males suggests that other factors, including estrogen, are needed. Consistent with this possibility it has been shown that progesterone administration to ovariectomized female monkeys and rats does not influence food intake (21,22).

The role of estrogen in food intake has been explored in female monkeys pretreated with progesterone. In these animals estradiol administration reduces food intake (19). Conversely, progesterone administration in monkeys chronically treated with estradiol does not change food intake (21). Thus, these animal studies suggest that the stimulatory effect of progesterone on food intake is due to its capacity to reduce the appetite suppressing effect of estrogen.

Research on the effects of estrogen and progesterone on the endogenous opioid system has lent further support to the role of these hormones in appetite. In the rat estradiol administration decreases sensitivity to naloxone, a specific opiate receptor antagonist which has been observed to decrease food intake under a variety of circumstances (22). The decrease in receptor response has been interpreted as one of the mechanisms by which estradiol treatment decreases food intake. The other possible mechanisms would involve a reduction in endogenous opioid peptides.

Estradiol administration in the rat also decreases the response to ketocyclazocine, a kappa agonist that stimulates feeding (23). Progesterone treatment reduces the estradiol effect on ketocyclazocine, thus providing further evidence of the interaction between these two hormones on appetite control. As previously mentioned, the idea of a "progesterone phase" and an "estrogen phase" of pregnancy, determined by the changing proportion in the plasma levels of these two hormones, fits well with the pattern of changes in food intake. During the first half of gestation maternal food intake would increase because of the antagonistic effect of progesterone on estrogen. During the second half the inhibition effect of estrogen would prevail. However, it would be overly simplistic to attribute the gestational changes in food intake solely to interactions between estrogen and progesterone (Fig. 7–3). The levels of other hormones known to influence food intake, such as insulin and glucagon, are also affected by pregnancy.

APPETITE CONTROL DURING LACTATION

The mechanisms responsible for the increased food intake observed in lactating animals have been explored in some detail in the rat (24). The following possibilities have been considered:

1. that nipple stimulation may convey signals into the hypothalamus capable of influencing hunger-satiety centers; and

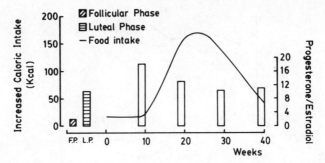

Figure 7-3. Changes in maternal calorie intake and progesterone: estradiol ratio during the course of pregnancy. Data on calorie intake adopted from (11). Data on plasma hormone levels during the menstrual cycle and pregnancy adopted from D. Talchinsky and K. J. Ryan, *Maternal-Fetal Endocrinology,* W. B. Saunders, Philadelphia, 1980.

2. that appetite is affected by the metabolic consequences of milk production and the consequent nutrient drain.

Ergocornine is an ergot alkaloid that inhibits prolactin secretion, and hence lactation, without disrupting maternal behavior. When injected into lactating rats, ergocornine causes a marked drop in food intake despite continuous suckling by the pups. This substance also decreases food intake in nonlactating rats, but the drop is minimal compared to that observed in lactating rats (Fig. 7-4). Thus, the data suggest that milk production per se, rather than nipple stimulation, is an important determinant of food intake in the rat. This conclusion is supported by the effect of galactophore ligation, which also inhibits milk production without interfering with suckling. After this operation lactating rats reduce their food intake although less than after engocornine injection.

Hormones seem to play no role in food intake during lactation. Prolactin administration alone or combined with hydrocortisone and oxytocin has no effect on the food intake of rats who had lactated for seven days and then weaned for ten days (24). Similarly, the effect of ovarian steroids has also been ruled out.

The mechanisms by which the "metabolic effect" of milk production ultimately influences the hunger-satiety mechanisms are unknown. There are observations suggesting that lactating rats

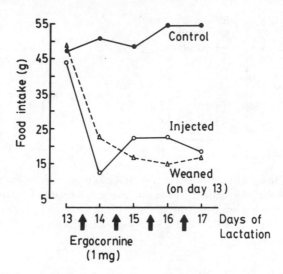

Figure 7–4 Maternal food intake in control, ergocornine injected, and weaned rats. Data from (24).

may have a reduced sensitivity to satiety factors (25). For example, a comparison of the effects of cholecystokinin (CCK) injection in lactating and nonlactating Zucker rats has revealed that this hormone, which causes a marked drop in food intake in virgin rats, does not alter food intake in lactating animals.

An increase in daily food intake can be accomplished by increasing meal frequencies or increasing meal size or both. Increases in meal size reflect reduced sensitivity to satiety factors. During lactation rats increase their daily food consumption by increasing meal size, rather than meal frequency. A similar phenomenon has been observed in the obese Zucker rat.

In summary, little is known about the mechanisms regulating food intake during pregnancy and lactation. The fragmentary information now available suggests that during pregnancy placental steroids may play an important role, but this possibility has not been experimentally tested. These steroids may affect appetite by interacting with the endogenous opioid system.

During lactation the main determinant of greater food con-

sumption seems to be the nutrient drain imposed by milk production. In contrast with pregnancy, hormones do not play a significant role. The metabolic or hormonal mediators that modulate
these food intake changes are unknown, but they seem to reduce
sensitivity to satiety factors. Overall, pregnancy and lactation appear to be two unique models of physiological hyperphagia which,
so far, have been neglected.

REFERENCES

1. A. W. Cripps and V. J. Williams, *Br. J. Nutr.*, **33**, 17 (1975).
2. *Recommended Dietary Allowances*, National Academy of Sciences, Washington, D.C., 1980.
3. E. B. Hook, *Am. J. Clin. Nutr.*, **31**, 1355 (1978).
4. G. Dickens and W. H. Trethowan, *J. Psychosom. Res.*, **15**, 259 (1971).
5. E. Payton, W. P. Crump, and P. Horton, *J. Am. Diet. Assn.*, **37**, 129 (1960).
6. C. M. Bruhn and R. M. Pangborn, *J. Am. Diet. Assn.*, **59**, 347 (1971).
7. R. Hansen and W. Langer, *Klin. Wschr.*, **14**, 1173 (1935).
8. L. Keith, H. Evenhouse, and A. Webster, *Obstet. Gynecol.*, **32**, 415 (1968).
9. J. E. Ansell and S. Wheby, *Va. Med. Q.*, **99**, 951 (1972).
10. K. M. Talkington, N. F. Gant, D. E. Scott, and J. A. Prichard, *Am. J. Obstet. Gynecol.*, **108**, 262 (1970).
11. V. Beal, *J. Am. Diet. Assn.*, **58**, 321 (1971).
12. G. Widlund, *Acta Obstet. Gynecol. Scand.*, **25**, Suppl I (1945).
13. F. E. Hytten and I. Leitch, *The Physiology of Human Pregnancy*, Blackwell Scient. Publ., Oxford, 1971 p. 415.
14. Ibid., p. 356.
15. R. L. Landau, J.A.M.A., **250**, 3323 (1983).
16. D. Talchinsky and C. J. Hobel, *Am. J. Obstetr. Gynecol.*, **17**, 884 (1973).
17. S. P. Dalvit, *Am. J. Clin. Nutr.*, **34**, 1811 (1981).
18. E. Hervey and G. R. Hervey, *J. Endocr.*, **37**, 361 (1967).
19. J. A. Czaja, *Physiol. Behav.*, **14**, 579 (1975).
20. R. L. Landau, D. M. Bergenstal, K. Lugibihil, and M. E. Kascht, *J. Clin. Endocrinol.*, **15**, 1194 (1955).
21. J. A. Czaja, *Physiol. Behav.*, **21**, 923 (1978).
22. G. R. Hervey and E. Hervey, *J. Endocrinol.*, **33**, 9 (1965).
23. J. E. Morley, A. S. Levine, M. Grace, J. Kneip, and B. A. Gosnell, *Physiol. Behav.*, **33**, 237 (1984).
24. A. S. Fleming, *Physiol. Behav.*, **17**, 841 (1976).
25. C. L. Mclanghlin, C. A. Baile, and S. R. Peikin, *Am. J. Physiol.*, **244**, E61 (1983).

8

Appetite in Anorexia of Cancer

ATHANASIOS THEOLOGIDES, M.D., Ph.D.
University of Minnesota Medical School and Hennepin County Medical
Center, Minneapolis, Minnesota

In clinical oncology anorexia implies a decrease in food intake, and in most patients with cancer such an implication is correct. However, some patients with malignant neoplastic diseases may maintain a good caloric intake, but at the same time complain about the palatability of the food and the lack of a pleasurable feeling with eating. They describe this negative experience as enjoying the food less than before, and, having developed food aversions, as certain foods having become unappealing and not tasting or smelling the same any more. They also complain frequently of rapid filling after a small quantity of food. So what a patient with cancer calls a loss of appetite might represent different experiences in different people. With time, of course, all these negative experiences lead to a fall in food intake.

For the purpose of this chapter, anorexia will imply a decreased food intake, and this will facilitate incorporation of laboratory data from experimental animals where appetite and anorexia cannot be evaluated otherwise. However, it should be emphasized that what is called loss of appetite and anorexia in cancer might represent a different symptom and a different phenomenon than anorexia nervosa, or loss of appetite with infections (hepatitis, AIDS, etc.) or other diseases. Actually cancer patients state that their anorexia is a different "feeling" than the loss of appetite they experienced with the "flu."

Anorexia is a common feature in cancer (1–3). It can be an early manifestation of the disease but as a rule it becomes a feature of the progressive cancer. As a presenting symptom its pathogenetic mechanism is clearly related to cancer because after a successful resection of the tumor or control of the disease with radiotherapy or chemotherapy the anorexia disappears. In contrast, later after the diagnosis and with a progressive disease additional factors contribute to the loss of appetite or to the worsening of the anorexia. Such factors are the psychological and emotional stress from the disease; pain, fever, and other symptoms; the anorexigenic effect of many drugs, such as analgesics or antibiotics; the anorexigenic and nausea inducing effect of radiotherapy and cancer chemotherapy; and complications of the treatment and of the disease, such as infections, hypercalcemia, and other metabolic abnormalities (4–6). All these contributory conditions may result in a significant fall of the total caloric intake, and also in major changes in the type of food consumed. Furthermore, there may be a change in the diurnal eating pattern, with patients frequently having a good appetite in the morning, enjoying a big breakfast, but then developing more and more anorexia as the day progresses.

The decreased food consumption contributes to the genesis of the syndrome of cachexia, which is characterized by marked anorexia, profound asthenia, anemia, relentless weight loss, and a decline of all body functions leading to death (7–14). The syndrome of cachexia basically is a metabolic derangement of the host as a remote effect of cancer. Alterations have been described in activity of enzymes, in carbohydrate, protein, and lipid metabolism, in metabolism of vitamins, trace elements, hormones, and in energy metabolism in general. It is of interest that many of the metabolic changes affect appetite and the resulting drop in food intake is responsible for a number of biochemical alterations. One such example is the abnormalities in zinc metabolism with cancer (3). However it should be stressed that patients with cancer may lose weight even with a good appetite and adequate food intake. This has become obvious as a result of the wide use of parenteral nutrition during oncologic management.

The anorexia is a source of great concern to the patient and relatives because it is taken as an ominous sign. Efforts are made to improve appetite and increase the caloric intake, hoping to reverse the consumptive process and the downhill course of the disease. But to increase food consumption in the presence of the cancer anorexia is a formidable, and usually unsuccessful, task.

INCIDENCE OF ANOREXIA IN CANCER

Animal Studies

Garattini and co-workers (15,16) reviewed studies on food intake during the growth of a variety of experimental tumors. They concluded that the majority of tumors induce a significant drop in food intake and in some the anorexia appears early, even when the tumor size is very small. In others it appears late, after the tumor reaches a certain size, and even in two sublines of the same tumor there may be a difference in when the anorexia appears (17). But the same tumor may also have a varying effect, producing more or less anorexia in comparable animals with even no anorexigenic effect in some animals in the group (15). It appears that the composition of the diet also plays a role in revealing the anorexia (15). On the other hand the status of the animal may influence the occurrence of anorexia; in one study obese mice became anorectic whereas lean mice became intensely polyphagic and the body weights changed accordingly (18).

Mordes and Rossini (19) described a rodent tumor system that appears suitable for the study of anorexia. They demonstrated that when the tumor was removed the food intake of the rat increased within 72 hours and the increase was sustained. Reimplantation of the tumor caused anorexia to occur. They also demonstrated that in parabiotic pairs of rats (common circulation) with tumor in one partner, the tumor free partner also experienced anorexia and weight loss. This observation suggested that the anorexia caused by the tumor is mediated by a circulating substance.

Human Studies

Although a loss of appetite is considered a common symptom in cancer there are not many studies documenting its incidence and severity in relation to the type of cancer, the location, and the organ involvement, or correlating it with a progression and a regression of the disease. A number of studies addressed some of these questions, usually with a small number of patients with a variety of cancers, at one time point or for relatively short periods and under different therapeutic regimens (20–26). There are, of course, major logistic, methodologic, psychosocial, and medical problems that make such long range studies very difficult. Needless to say, long term studies with significant numbers of patients, correlating the anorexia and the qualitative and quantitative changes in food intake to progression and posttherapeutic regression of cancer, may assist in our understanding of the pathogenesis of cancer anorexia.

Any such studies face the problem of controls. When normal control subjects are used as reference for adequacy of food intake the problem is that there is a wide range of what is considered adequate or "normal" caloric intake. When a period before the diagnosis of cancer is used as a baseline for the patient's intake the problem is that the data are based on recollection. Usually the changes are gradual and the patient may underestimate the intake before the diagnosis and minimize the magnitude of the change. Intake data collected while the patient is in the hospital are more objective, but they have pitfalls related to the environment and unappealing hospital meals.

Hoffman (20) reported anorexia in 8.4% of male and 11.6% of female patients with cancer. We reported (21) anorexia in 15.3% of patients admitted to the hospital for initiation of chemotherapy because of metastases. Another 25% of our patients complained of "easy filling" or early satiety despite a good initial appetite. Willox and co-workers reported an incidence of 43% in their study (22).

In our study (21) the food intake of patients with cancer was evaluated at four time periods:

1. before the diagnosis of cancer,
2. at the time of diagnosis,
3. at the time of the dissemination of the disease, and

4. during the first hospitalization for chemotherapy or radiotherapy.

Patients included in the study met the following criteria. It was
their first admission to our institution and the original diagnosis
of cancer was made within the previous three years. This period
was selected arbitrarily for the patients to be able to make a rather
accurate recollection of food intake prior to the diagnosis. During
the previous three years the patient should not have followed any
medically or otherwise prescribed or self-imposed diet. During the
hospitalization they should have been on a normal diet. Patients
were excluded from the study on the basis of a number of criteria
(21).

During the study period 439 patients were admitted to the medical oncology service and 39 met the criteria and were evaluated.
These patients had a variety of solid tumors or lymphomas at an
advanced state but had had no prior chemotherapy or radiotherapy. The questionnaire for the dietary intake recorded intake and
nutritional information for the first three periods, including
changes in appetite, food cravings, food aversions and intolerances, and weight changes. For period 4 the caloric intake and
distribution in the hospital were recorded for a minimum of three
and a maximum of five days prior to chemotherapy or radiotherapy. The intake for period 1 was compared to the 1965–1966 national survey of food and nutrient intake to determine whether
there was any significant difference between the population as a
whole and the patients studied.

All 39 patients were initially analyzed as one group. The patients then were arbitrarily divided into two groups; one group
(18 patients) who from period 1 to period 3 had a weight loss of
greater than 10% of their usual weight and another group (21 patients) with less than 10% loss of weight or weight gain. Five of the
18 and one of the 21 complained of decreased appetite. Of the 18
patients with weight loss ten had 300 calories or more decreased
intake from period 1 to period 3 (range 300–2,241). Five of these
ten reported that their appetite was "still good" but the decreased
intake was due to "easy filling." Of the 21 patients without weight

loss, four had a similar drop in calorie intake from period 1 to period 3. The decrease was usually in all three macronutrients. There was no correlation between oligophagia and wasting, but weight loss with unchanged caloric intake and stable weight with decreased intake were also observed. A few patients without anorexia and with a calorie intake within the national average for their weight, age, and sex and within the recommended allowances for maintenance of good nutrition in healthy persons had significant weight loss. Patients with decreased intake maintained their food preferences and meal patterns. No food cravings or intolerances were observed (21).

Costa and his co-workers (23,24), demonstrated that male cancer patients ate significantly less than their control subjects. In a small but homogeneous subset of male lung cancer patients, anorexia and weight loss were found to be unrelated and the anorexia could not solely account for the weight loss observed. Surprisingly the small group of female patients maintained their food consumption.

DeWys and co-workers (25) studied caloric intake in 89 cancer patients who recorded diet diaries. Twenty-five percent had caloric intake below their calculated basal energy expenditure (BEE) and an additional 45% had caloric intake between 1.0 and 1.4 times BEE.

Recently Lindsey and Piper (26) observed that ten male study subjects had a drop in spontaneous food intake in the first five months following the diagnosis of a small cell lung carcinoma. The decline in the mean caloric intake at 18 weeks was 502 Kcal per day and such an oral intake was less than adequate for any activity beyond the basal state. Decreased intake could account for most of the weight loss observed in the subjects. They observed a relative consistency over time in the percent distribution of fat intake and more variability in the protein and carbohydrate intake; an increase in the percent of carbohydrate at the expense of protein was the most notable change. Burke and co-workers (27) also reported such a decline in protein and caloric intake in those cancer patients who lost weight. In our study (21) in the majority of patients the decrease in calorie intake was comparable for the three macronutrients and only occasionally were there discrepancies such as increased consumption of one nutrient and decreased consumption of another. Various combinations were observed with no particular trend. More clinical studies are needed in loss of appetite and anorexia in cancer.

FOOD AVERSIONS

The patient with cancer who complains that he does not "feel like eating" occasionally atrributes this to the development of dislikes for certain foods that were very appealing and palatable before. Such food aversions have been studied mainly by Bernstein's group (28–35). The aversions may be interpreted as anorexia and they may contribute to decreased food intake. They have been compared to those developing during pregnancy (36).

Usually aversions to certain foods develop in response to unpleasant symptoms and temporary sickness associated with chemotherapy or radiotherapy. But there is evidence also that the growth of a tumor itself may be responsible for the development of food aversions by inducing some chronic symptoms or some metabolic changes in the host. The development of such food aversions associated with a tumor growth has been supported by experimental work in animals demonstrating different effects in different tumors (34,35). Animals with Leydig tumors developed strong aversions to the specific diet they had eaten after tumor implant but animals with Walker-256 tumor did not develop any (34,35). The identification of the physiologic changes responsible for the formation of aversions caused by tumors is a challenging problem.

Although the patient may become conditioned to reject the food on seeing it the rejection usually comes after smelling or tasting it, and this suggests that there are alterations in perception in these senses during cancer growth.

Abnormalities in Taste Perception

Patients occasionally complain that the "turning away" from certain foods results from these foods' not tasting the same any more.

To study this phenomenon a number of investigators evaluated taste thresholds during the course of cancer. Thresholds for the four taste qualities have been compared between cancer patients and people without cancer, with or without treatments (37–42). Compared to control groups, in cancer patients recognition thresholds have been observed to be increased for salt and sweet and increased or decreased for sour and bitter taste. For instance, in one study with a mixed group of cancer patients, together with an increased threshold for sweetness (sucrose) there was a decreased threshold for bitterness (urea) while no changes were found in the threshold for sourness (hydrochloric acid) and saltiness (sodium chloride). The increased threshold for sweet and the decreased threshold for bitter were observed in about 25% and 14%, respectively, of cancer patients. Radiotherapy and chemotherapy also cause changes in taste sensation (44,45).

The controversial results, to a certain extent, are attributed to the types of cancer and the extent of disease in patients in the different groups studied and the variety of concomitant treatments. A relation of zinc deficiency to taste changes and appetite loss also remains controversial (43). But it is generally accepted that changes in taste perceptions occur in patients with cancer and as a result certain foods suddenly have less pleasurable effect. One observation that is intriguing is that with a restoration of a nutritional deficit with intravenous hyperalimentation taste function and appetite may improve (46).

Abnormalities in Odor Perception

Although changes in the sense of smell in cancer patients have been suspected, studies have not been reported prior to 1980 on the role of odor perception in the development of food aversions and decreased food intake in such patients. In 1980 we reported the first such study (47,48).

The primary objective of the study was to determine whether cancer patients with food aversions perceived the pleasantness or intensity of common food odors differently from cancer patients who did not experience food aversions or differently from control subjects. A second objective was to correlate the odor testing data and the data from the questionnaire on food preferences and smell or taste changes for foods. The study also sought to determine any relationship between the presence of food aversions, decreased appetite, weight loss, or early satiety and the type of cancer or the administration of chemotherapy.

In this study 133 patients with cancer and 50 healthy control subjects judged the pleasantness of ten common food odors. The food odors tested were corn, green beans, blueberry, lemon, coffee, chocolate, ham, pork, roast beef, and chicken. The patients also completed a questionnaire on food likes or dislikes, recent smell or taste changes, development of food aversions, weight loss, decreased appetite, and early satiety. Chocolate, pork, roast beef, and chicken odors were significantly less pleasant for patients with food aversions than for control subjects. Ham, pork, and roast beef odors were significantly less pleasant for patients with food aversions than for patients without food aversions. More patients with aversions than control subjects or patients without food aversions reported recent smell and taste changes for most of the ten foods in the sample set. Roast beef was the only food on the questionnaire rated significantly less pleasant by patients with aversions than control subjects or patients without food aversions. There were no significant correlations between the testing odor hedonic scores and the questionnaires hedonic scores for any of the ten foods. More patients with than without aversions had weight loss, decreased appetite, and early satiety. Patients receiving chemotherapy did not have a significantly greater incidence of aversions, weight loss, decreased appetite, or early satiety than patients not receiving chemotherapy. The type of cancer did not appear to have any relation to the development of food aversions, but the number of patients with any one type of cancer was rather small (47).

In summary, patients with cancer develop aversions to certain foods and it appears that alterations in the hedonic food effects on the sense of smell and taste play a role in their development leading to a decreased food intake. Red meats, coffee, and chocolate are the foods most frequently mentioned by cancer patients. But the actual contribution of learned aversions to the total anorexia picture remains unknown (34).

EARLY SATIETY

A common complaint in patients with cancer is an early satiety, with the patient feeling hungry before the meal but becoming full and anorectic after a few bites. The physiology of normal satiety remains poorly understood so it is not surprising that the pathogenesis of early satiety in cancer is totally unknown. This symptom may be responsible for a significant drop in intake and in one experimental system the oligophagia was entirely attributable to premature satiety (49).

DeWys (50) considered early satiety to be the result of three effects of cancer on the gastrointestinal tract:

1. decreased production of digestive secretions leading to delayed digestion,
2. atrophic changes in the mucosa of the small intestine, and
3. wasting of the muscular wall of the stomach and delayed emptying.

A tumor associated gastroparesis resulting in a delayed gastric emptying has been demonstrated (51).

However it appears that early satiety is a more generalized manifestation of cancer and may have a pathogenetic mechanism comparable to that of the cancer anorexia (3). But this remains a hypothesis.

ASTHENIA

Asthenia is one of the most prominent features of advanced cancer and it involves a decrease in motor and mental capabilities that is difficult to quantitate (52). This systemic debility is characterized physically by generalized weakness, loss of strength, and an easy fatigability of the muscles (52). The marked weakness and easy fatigability may affect food intake because eating becomes an exhausting process. The asthenia may contribute to the decreased food consumption per meal.

PATHOGENESIS OF ANOREXIA IN CANCER

Although significant progress has been made in our understanding of the genesis of hunger and satiety and the signals that initiate and the mechanisms that control food intake in normal persons, the pathogenesis of the anorexia in cancer patients remains unknown. Recent reviews have discussed the phenomena and the evolution of theories for the physiology of control of food intake with a particular emphasis on the function of neural and humoral signals (53–55). With the introduction of any new hypothesis on regulation, the theory was tested in tumor bearing animals in an effort to explain their anorexia.

The old dual center theory for the central regulatory system for hunger and satiety provided anatomical regions in the brain responsible for the control of feeding. The ventromedial nuclei of the hypothalamus represented the satiety centers and the lateral nuclei the feeding centers, with higher regions exerting modifying influences. The function of these brain centers during distant cancer growth has been investigated. When the Walker tumor was transplanted into rats previously rendered polyphagic by destruction of the ventromedial hypothalamic areas, the cancer anorexia appeared and the food intake began to decline 15 days after the transplantation and eventually reached very low levels (56). There was no evidence for any malfunction of these distinct centers. Gradually the earlier concepts of the dual brain centers for the regulation of hunger and satiety have been replaced by the concept of brain receptor mechanisms at various sites, with biochemically different systems for the onset and termination of eating.

The alimentary tract regulation with the oropharyngeal region and the stomach metering the quantity of food eaten on a meal-to-meal basis might be altered during tumor growth. Morrison (57) demonstrated that growth of Walker-256 carcinosarcoma depressed the hyperingestive response of rats to dilution of food with nonnutritive bulk. In view of the observation that satiety induces gut peptides (see below) this theory needs more testing in tumor bearing animals. Especially in view of bombesin and somatostatin mediating satiety messages from the stomach and the production of comparable peptides by cancer this theory becomes more exciting.

The thermostatic regulation theory stimulated the search for substances produced by the cancer that could uncouple the oxidative phosphorylation and result in an increased heat liberation. This could explain the anorexia of cancer and also an energy wasting and negative energy balance in the host. Substances were found in tumor extracts and in the serum of sarcoma bearing rats that could uncouple the oxidative phosphorylation of normal liver mitochondria in vitro (58,59). However there are no observations demonstrating an in vivo alteration in the energy yielding and coupling mechanisms in tumor bearing hosts to explain the anorexia on the basis of the thermostatic theory. When anorectic tumor bearing rats were placed in a cold environment, they increased their food intake temporarily, but the anorexia reappeared subsequently (60). It was concluded by Stevenson and his co-workers that initially the demand for heat production to maintain homeostasis was a stronger stimulus and that it overshadowed the anorexigenic effect of malignant growth. In another study Morrison (61) observed that the cold-specific feeding response to cold exposure was depressed by 30% by the presence of tumor. The fact remains that there are major perturbations in the metabolism and energy balance in tumor free tissue of the cancer host, but it is unclear if these changes contribute to the genesis of cancer anorexia.

The glucostatic regulation hypothesis was also tested in animals and patients with cancer. Patients with cancer have a high incidence of diabetic glucose tolerance curve (62). Although their fasting blood sugar does not differ significantly from that of tumor free controls, they have a markedly lower than normal rate of disappearance of the intravenously given glucose (63,64). These aberrations of carbohydrate metabolism are comparable to those of a subclinical diabetes and if anything, one would expect an increased appetite as in diabetes mellitus. In the cancer bearing host, liver and muscle glycogen content declines, gluconeogenesis is increased, and Cori cycle activity increases (65), but such biochemical changes in carbohydrate metabolism are not known to affect appetite through brain glucoreceptors. Cancer patients with marked lactic acidemia have been described but there is no evidence that high levels of lactic acid are responsible for anorexia in most of them. The polyphagia induced by insulin is present to the same extent before and after Walker-256 transplantation, indicating that "glucose receptors" for feeding are not altered during tumor growth (57). If and how abnormalities in carbohydrate metabolism in cancer affect appetite remain unknown.

With the postulation of a lipostatic mechanism for the regulation of food intake (66) a circulating factor was sought that could be in a dynamic equilibrium with the total fat in the body and could inform brain regions for a long term regulation of fat stores. A tumor, by producing such factors, could influence the central regulatory mechanism of the host and could induce the anorexia (2). However no such substances could be determined. In one study there was a good correlation between the onset of anorexia and the increase in free fatty acids in fed tumor bearing animals (67). The meaning of this observation remains obscure, although again one could postulate that free fatty acids play a role in cancer anorexia. There is no experimental evidence of changes during cancer growth to suggest that abnormalities of osmoreceptors are responsible for the anorexia of cancer.

As for the regulation of hunger and satiety by amino acids, relevant to cancer are the observations that the free amino acid pattern of the blood and tissues of the hosts are altered during the growth of the tumor. These alterations are probably primary effects of cancer and less a secondary result of the malnutrition. In support of this is the finding that the total amino acid nitrogen in the blood of cancer patients is elevated, in contrast to the starving person in whom it is decreased (2). In pair feeding experiments, when the control animal was given the quantity of food consumed by the tumor bearing one the day before, decreased plasma levels of serine, glycine, aspartate, and hydroxyproline were found in tumor bearing rats only and not in the pair fed controls (73). Abnormalities of amino acid patterns in the blood and their metabolic consequences probably are contributory factors to the genesis of anorexia in cancer (68–75). Amino acid concentrations and profiles in different parts of the brain might even be more important in view of the fact that some act as neurotransmitters or are precursors in neurotransmitter synthesis and this way may influence feeding behavior (73,75). The mechanism of amino acid regulation needs more study in cancer anorexia.

As for the possibility of an abnormality in hormonal regulation of food intake in patients with cancer, a number of hormonal imbalances have been observed in such patients but nothing that can be incriminated as inducing anorexia. For instance, the production of ACTH and adrenal corticosteroids is increased (76,77). With this high blood level of corticosteroids one would expect increased appetite rather than anorexia. There is direct evidence that insulin pharmacologically induces a polyphagic response in rats bearing Walker-256 carcinosarcoma (see below). There is recent evidence that estrogens play a role in the genesis of anorexia in one tumor system. Mordes and co-workers concluded that the circulating substance responsible for LTW(m) tumor induced anorexia in male rats is likely to be an estrogenic steroid (78). With the reported interrelations between gut and brain peptides and hormones, this area is open for research in cancer anorexia.

Recently the interest in food intake regulation has shifted to the role of the peptidergic and monoaminergic systems (53–55, 79–84) and also their modulation by a variety of nutrients and of hormones from the classical endocrine system (55). It appears that there is a peripheral and a central satiety system. In the peripheral system gastrointestinal hormones released during the passage of food contribute to the genesis of satiety. Cholecystokinin and somatostatin clearly appear to be the main satiety agents, but other peptides under investigation include bombesin, gastric-releasing peptide, glucagon calcitonin, and thyrotropin-releasing hormone (55).

The picture is more confusing for neurotransmitters, which play a role in the central regulation of hunger and satiety (55). Satiety centers in the ventromedial hypothalamus are thought to be under serotonergic influence, with serotonic agonists producing anorexia (53). An alpha-adrenergic system may excite feeding by inhibiting part of the ventromedial hypothalamus satiety center, and norepinephrine injected into the medial hypothalamus produces feeding through such an effect. Depletion of norepinephrine with a dopamine beta hydroxylase inhibitor reduces food intake (53). Alpha agonists produce feeding drive by stimulation of the release of gamma-aminobutyric acid in the ventro-medial hypothalamus (55).

A beta-adrenergic system is thought to cause satiety by inhibiting the classical ventrolateral hypothalamus. For instance, inhibition of food intake by the hungry rat occurs when isoproterenol, a beta-adrenergic drug, is injected into the lateral hypothalamus. Beta-adrenergic blockers such as propranolol stimulate food intake. Dopamine agonists help restore food ingestion (53).

The central injection of beta-endorphin enhances feeding (85) and naloxone reduces feeding in most but not in all species (55). In some instances food intake may be initiated by a tonic dopaminergic-opioid mechanism in the region of the lateral hypothalamus (55). Dynorphin and other kappa-agonists initiate feeding (55). A mu-opioid may play a role in producing anorexia (84), but at present which of the observed experimental effects are physiologic and which are pharmacologic is unclear.

Some of these new systems and agents in the regulation of food intake have been evaluated recently in tumor bearing animals; the results of the studies remain preliminary and in many respects controversial. However this area will see increasing research activity in an effort to elucidate the pathogenesis of cancer anorexia and early satiety. A number of the initial studies will be reviewed here.

Krause and co-workers suggested that the central serotonergic system involving tryptophan and its indole neurotransmitter metabolites is deranged in neoplastic diseases. They observed that rats bearing intramuscular (IM) Walker-256 tumors exhibited decreased eating six days after tumor induction which kept increasing in severity until the death of the animal. Biochemical analysis of the brains of these rats indicated increased levels of tryptophan and 5-hydroxyindole acetic acid. The absence of such changes in rats that were pair fed the same amount of food as the tumor bearing ones suggested that the changes were not merely a result of malnutrition. These changes appeared to be secondary to an increased level of free tryptophan in the plasma. They postulated that such changes in central neurotransmitter metabolism may contribute to the genesis of anorexia in cancer (86,87). In other experiments they observed the increase in whole brain tryptophan, serotonin, and 5-hydroxyindole acetic acid in another line of anorexia producing tumor and concluded that the increased serotonin activity is a general phenomenon (88).

Subsequently, to more fully investigate the role of brain serotonin (5-HT) in cancer anorexia, they employed acute intraventricular injections of parachlorophenylalanine (PCPA), an inhibitor of tryptophan hydroxylase. Significant anorexia had developed six days after the induction (IM) of Walker-256 carcinomas in saline treated rats. Although tumor bearing rats treated with PCPA ate less than the PCPA injected controls, by day seven their feeding response was significantly greater than that of saline treated tumor bearing rats on days five, six and seven. The PCPA treatment had no significant effect on food intake in nontumor bearing rats. Brain serotonin, 5-hydroxyindole acetic acid, and norepinephrine levels were decreased in PCPA treated rats. The investigators concluded that although these data may provide some support for a serotonergic mediation of cancer anorexia, additional mechanisms are clearly involved (89).

Additional work from the same laboratory raised significant doubts about the importance of the indoleamine system in the etiology of cancer anorexia. The anorectic effects of cancer (Walker-256) were investigated in immature female rats that had been depleted of brain serotonin (5-HT) by the intracisternal injection of 5,7-dihydroxytryptamine (5,7-DHT) or the systemic injection of parachloroamphetamine (PCA). Although both 5,7-DHT and PCA significantly reduced brain concentration of 5-HT and 5-HIAA by approximately 50% no effects on the onset or severity of the anorectic response to cancer were observed (90). Neither compound affected eating in nontumor bearing control animals. Therefore these data did not support increased brain 5-HT activity as a primary mediator of cancer anorexia, but the authors concluded that a role of monoamines may eventually be established in cancer anorexia (90). The role acquired new significance after observations of regional brain changes in tryphophan metabolism in cancer bearing animals (91).

Nichols and co-workers demonstrated that tumor bearing rats with a 40% reduction in food intake had higher nighttime plasma free tryptophan and regional 5-hydroxyindole acetic acid levels than their pair fed malnourished controls. No significant difference in tryptophan, serotonin, or 5-hydroxyindole acetic acid levels was detected between pair fed and tumor bearing rats exhibiting only a 20% reduction of nighttime food intake. These results indicated that increased plasma free tryptophan and elevated serotonin metabolism may not be the initial dysfunction responsible for nocturnal anorexia. However, it may contribute to the decreasing nocturnal food intake in severely anorectic tumor rats (92). Previous work from their laboratory (93) showed a relationship between attenuated 2-deoxy-D-glucose induced polyphasia and depleted daytime hypothalamic norepinephrine levels in Walker-256 tumor bearing rats. However, more recent results from the same laboratory indicated that the anorexia is not due to depletion of central catecholamines (94). Obviously the role of central catecholamines in the cancer anorexia remains controversial at this point and more research is needed.

Cholecystokinin was accepted as a satiety signal after the demonstration that systemic administration decreased eating in rats and elicited a behavioral pattern of satiety (95,96). The interaction of cholecystokinin induced oligophagia with cancer anorexia was investigated within both acute (Walker-256 carcinosarcoma) and chronic (methylcholanthrene induced sarcoma) animal models of cancer anorexia (97). Cholecystokinin octapeptide (CCK-8) effectively reduced feeding for at least one hour in experimental and control animals. However, at a variety of doses both before and after the development of anorexia this peptide was no more effective in inducing oligophagia in tumor bearing rats than in nontumor bearing control animals (97). Therefore these observations did not support a role of cholecystokinin in the mediation of experimental cancer anorexia, since no synergism of CCK-8 induced oligophagia with the anorexia was observed. The absence of synergism of CCK induced oligophagia with the anorexia of cancer immediately before each onset suggests that changes in endogenous CCK levels are not primarily responsible for cancer anorexia (97).

In another study plasma and brain concentrations of CCK were determined by radioimmunoassay in anorectic tumor bearing rats (98). Plasma concentrations of immunoreactive CCK were not significantly altered in either an aggressive Walker-256

carcinosarcoma or a more slow growing methylcholanthrene induced sarcoma animal model of cancer anorexia (98). Levels of
immunoreactive CCK were significantly reduced in the hypothalamus and cerebral cortex of animals bearing the methylcholanthrene sarcoma during both mild and severe anorexia. These data
demonstrate that elevations in immunoreactive CCK are not a major factor in the etiology of early satiety and anorexia in cancer.
The authors raised the question that if brain CCK is involved in
satiety then tumor bearing rats may be attempting to compensate
for their anorexia by down regulating CCK production, which is
responsible for the observed lower levels in the brain.

The area of peptidergic regulation of appetite and possible perturbations with cancer is an exciting field for research in the future. The present knowledge on the role of monoamines, opioids,
and brain and gut peptides in the control of feeding has been
reviewed and discussed critically by Morley and co-workers (99)
and by Hoebel (100) and many of the reviewed studies could be
repeated in tumor bearing animals.

Hypothesis on the Pathogenesis

There are numerous peripheral and central anatomical monitor
sites for the normal control of food intake, with the hypothalamus
representing the main computing and commanding area. There
is also a plethora of signals and messages informing these sites.
Various perturbations in this complex mechanism may produce
different types of anorexia that cannot be distinguished at present
at the pathophysiologic or clinical level. This makes it reasonable
to propose that in cancer too there might be different types and
different mechanisms of loss of appetite and anorexia, depending
on the type of cancer, the location and organ involvement, and
the alterations in the biochemistry of host tissues.

There is good evidence that the growth of cancer is associated
with the appearance of substances in the blood and urine, substances that can induce anorexia when injected into other animals
(2,19,101). In the past we advanced the hypothesis that these substances were peptides (4) released by the cancer or secondarily

from host tissues. Such peptides could be called collectively "anorexins" and could act both peripherally and centrally. It is almost a universal phenomenon for cancers to produce peptides and other small molecules, most probably as a result of depression of various genomes (102). The "anorexins" could represent such peptides.

Recently there is an increasing interest in "cachectins" (103,104), substances that might play a key role in the development of weight loss and the cachexia of cancer. Such work might stimulate the search for "anorexins."

Cancer peptides may also be responsible for the alterations in the senses of smell and taste. There is already evidence that substance P and opioids play a role in modulating taste perception in healthy persons (55).

THE MANAGEMENT OF ANOREXIA

The loss of appetite in the cancer patient and the decrease in food intake and malnutrition that follow adversely affect the quality of life and the tolerance to oncologic therapy and increase the incidence and severity of complications of the disease and of the treatment. Ultimately they adversely affect the survival. For this reason efforts were made to increase the caloric intake through different dietetic approaches and other means (105,106). However, there are no orexigenic agents capable of stimulating appetite in the anorectic cancer patient.

Cyproheptidine, an antihistamine-antiserotonin agent, showed an appetite stimulating effect in man (15). It has been used in cancer patients in some studies (15,107,108), but unfortunately the results are limited and insufficiently controlled to permit any conclusions.

In tumor bearing rats in an early stage of cachexia insulin increased food intake and host weight (total body weight minus tumor weight) (109). When daily insulin administration was started at an early stage of tumor growth and continued until death there was again significant enhancement of food intake and host weight. But survival time was slightly reduced in tumor bearing rats treated with long term insulin although there was no stimulation of tumor growth with insulin (109).

Pharmacologic doses of adrenocorticosteroids do increase the appetite in anorectic cancer patients but this effect is short lived and it is associated with their side effects. In a double-blind cross-over trial prednisolone 5 mg three times a day was given for two weeks, and for a third week when the doses were reduced. Patients with a variety of solid tumors were included in the study, but gastrointestinal cancers were the most common. Some also received concomitant chemotherapy. Prednisolone was significantly better than placebo in improving appetite in patients with cancer in the short term; this improvement was seen also when patients who had been taking placebo crossed over to receive prednisolone. However there was a major placebo effect, confirming also a psychological factor for anorexia in some of the patients. When taking prednisolone the patients showed a trend towards increased intake and a significant increase in well being (22). A beneficial effect on appetite was demonstrated in another study in terminal cancer patients (110). But because of the transient benefit and the side effects corticosteroids are not routinely used for that purpose.

With the consideration that an increased brain tryptophan level, resulting in an increased serotonin synthesis and turnover, may contribute to anorexia, efforts were made to influence food intake by decreasing brain tryptophan. Increased brain tryptophan is presumably due to decreased binding of tryptophan to plasma albumin as a result of competition with nonesterified fatty acids, whose level is increased in cancer. An increase in plasma free tryptophan augments tryptophan transport into the brain (111). These investigators reasoned that if this hypothesis is correct, increasing the concentration of plasma branched chain amino acids (BCAA) would be expected to increase competition with tryptophan for transport into the brain and delay the emergence of anorexia. By adding BCAA to the diet of tumor bearing rats they delayed the onset of tumor related anorexia (111). It is questionable if these observations will have any clinical relevance.

The appearance of anorexia with zinc deficiency is well known and it is not mediated by changes in plasma amino acid concentrations, but the zinc deficiency per se directly affects appetite (112).

Recent work suggests that abnormalities in endogenous opiate regulation of appetite may play a role in the anorexia of zinc deficiency (113). The fact remains that patients with cancer demonstrated abnormalities in zinc metabolism, with low serum zinc levels and high urinary zinc excretion (114). Although patients with anorexia nervosa have been reported to respond to zinc administration (115,116), at this point there is no convincing evidence that zinc supplementation can improve the anorexia in cancer.

At present there are no known physiologic or pharmacologic means to stimulate the appetite in the cancer patient. Only a successful surgical, radiotherapeutic, or chemotherapeutic treatment reverses the anorexia.

REFERENCES

1. A. Theologides, *Cancer,* **29,** 484 (1972).
2. A. Theologides, *Ann. N.Y. Acad. Sci.,* **230,** 14 (1974).
3. A. Theologides, *Cancer Bull.,* **34**(4), 140 (1982).
4. A. Theologides, *Am. J. Clin. Nutr.,* **29,** 552 (1976).
5. J. C. B. Holland, J. Rowland, and M. Plumb, *Cancer Res.,* **37,** 2425 (1977).
6. W. D. DeWys, *Cancer Res.,* **37,** 2354 (1977).
7. A. Theologides, "Cancer Cachexia," in M. Winick, Ed., *Nutrition and Cancer,* Wiley, New York, 1977, p. 75.
8. J. Gold, *Ann. N.Y. Acad. Sci.,* **230,** 103 (1974).
9. G. Costa, *Cancer Res.,* **37,** 2327 (1977).
10. J. C. Hall, *Biomedicine,* **30,** 287 (1979).
11. J. F. Williams, K. I. Matthaei, M. Graham, et al., *Cancer Forum,* **21,** 118 (1980).
12. A. J. Strain, G. C. Easty, and A. M. Neville, *J.N.C.I.,* **64,** 217 (1980).
13. Y. Kondo, K. Sato, Y. Ueyama, et al., *Cancer Res.,* **41,** 2912 (1981).
14. R. I. C. Wesdorp, R. Krause, and M. F. Von Meyenfeldt, *Br. J. Surg.,* **70,** 352 (1983).
15. S. Garattini, A. Bizzi, M. G. Donelli, A. Guiatani, R. Samanin, and F. Spreafico, *Cancer Treat. Rev.,* **7** (3), 115 (1980).
16. S. Garattini and A. Guiatani, *Cancer Treat. Rep.,* **65** (Suppl 5), 23 (1981).
17. A. Guiatani, P. D. Torre, L. Morasca, C. Pintus, and I. Bartosek, *Tumori,* **69,** 1 (1983).
18. C. I. Thompson, J. W. Kreider, and D. L. Margules, *Physiol. Behav.,* **32,** 935 (1984).
19. J. P. Mordes and A. A. Rossini, *Science,* **213,** 565 (1981).
20. F. L. Hoffman. *Cancer and Diet,* Williams and Wilkins, Baltimore, 1937, p. 463.
21. A. Theologides, J. Ehlert, and B. J. Kennedy, *Minn. Med.,* **50,** 526 (1976).

22. J. C. Willox, J. Corr, J. Shaw, M. Richardson, K. C. Calman, and M. Drennan, *Br. Med. J.*, **288**, 27 (1984).

23. G. Costa, P. Bewley, M. Aragon, and J. Siebold, *Cancer Treat. Rep.*, **65** (Suppl 5), 3 (1981).

24. G. Costa, W. W. Lane, R. G. Vincent, J. A. Siebold, M. Aragon, and P. T. Bewley, *Nutr. Cancer*, **2**, 98 (1981).

25. W. D. DeWys, G. Costa, and R. Henkin, *Cancer Treat. Rep.*, **65** (suppl 5), 49 (1981).

26. A. M. Lindsey and B. F. Piper, *Nutr. Cancer*, **7**, 65 (1985).

27. M. Burke, E. L. Bryson, and A. E. Kark, *Br. Med. J.*, **26**, 211 (1980).

28. I. L. Bernstein, *Science*, **200**, 1302 (1978).

29. I. L. Bernstein and M. M. Webster, *Physiol. Behav.*, **25**, 363 (1980).

30. I. L. Bernstein and R. A. Sigmundi, *Science*, **209**, 416 (1980).

31. J. C. Smith and J. T. Blumsack, *Cancer Treat. Rep.*, **65** (Suppl 5), 37 (1981).

32. I. L. Bernstein and I. D. Bernstein, *Cancer Treat. Rep.*, **65** (Suppl 5), 43, (1981).

33. I. L. Bernstein, *Cancer Res.*, (Suppl) **42**, 715 (1982).

34. I. L. Bernstein, *Ann. N.Y. Acad. Sci.*, **443**, 365 (1985).

35. I. L. Bernstein and D. P. Fenner, *J. Intake Res.*, **4**, 79, 1983.

36. T. B. Brewin, *Lancet*, **2**, 907 (1980).

37. I. T. Abasov, *Sov. Med.*, **25**, 47 (1961).

38. W. D. DeWys and K. Walters, *Cancer*, **36**, 1888 (1974).

39. J. A. S. Carson and A. Gormican, *J. Am. Dietet. Assn.*, **70**, 361 (1977).

40. R. I. Henkin, *Ann. N.Y. Acad. Sci.*, **300**, 383 (1977).

41. D. Gorshein, *Cancer*, **39**, 1700 (1977).

42. L. R. Williams and M. H. Cohen, *Am. J. Clin. Nutr.*, **31**, 122 (1978).

43. T. A. Sontag, *Dissert. Abst. Internat.*, **41** (12) 4467B (1981).

44. T. B. Brewin, *Clin. Radiol.*, **33**, 471 (1982).

45. N. H. Mulder, J. M. Smit, W. M. I. Kreumer, J. Bouman, D. T. Sleijfer, W. Veeger, and H. S. Koops, *Oncology*, **40**, 36 (1983).

46. J. E. Russ and W. D. DeWys, *Arch. Int. Med.*, **138**, 799 (1978).

47. S. S. Neilsen, A. Theologides, and Z. M. Vickers, *Clin. Nutr.*, **33**, 2253 (1980).

48. Z. M. Vickers, S. S. Nielsen, and A. Theologides, *Minn. Med.*, **64**, 277 (1981).

49. S. D. Morrison, *Cancer Res.*, **44**, 1041 (1984).

50. W. D. DeWys, *Cancer*, **43**, 2013 (1979).

51. K. Shivshanker, R. W. Bennetts, and T. P. Haynie, *Gastroenterology*, **80**, 1283 (1981).

52. A. Theologides, *Am. J. Med.*, **73**, 1 (1982).

53. J. E. Morley, *Life Sci.*, **27**, 355 (1980).

54. H. R. Kissileff and T. B. VanItallie, *Ann. Rev. Nutr.*, **2**, 371 (1982.

55. J. E. Morley and A. S. Levine, *Med. J. Austral.*, **142** (Suppl) 511 (1985).

56. P. Baillie, F. K. Millar, and A. W. Platt, *Am. J. Physiol.*, **209**, 293 (1965).

57. S. D. Morrison, *Cancer Res.*, **33**, 526 (1973).

58. T. M. Devlin and M. P. Pruss, *Fed. Proc.*, **17**, 211 (1958).

59. G. Nanni and A. Casu, *Experientia*, **17**, 402 (1961).

60. J. A. F. Stevenson, B. M. Box, and R. B. Wright, *Can. J. Biol. Physiol.*, **41**, 531 (1961).

61. S. D. Morrison, *Cancer Res.*, **42**, 490 (1982).

62. A. S. Glicksman and R. W. Rawson, *Cancer*, **9**, 1127 (1956).

63. P. A. Marks and J. S. Bishop, *Proc. Am. Assn. Cancer Res.*, **2**, 131 (1956).

64. P. A. Marks and J. S. Bishop, *Cancer Res.*, **2**, 228 (1957).

65. J. Singh, M. R. Grigor, and M. P. Thompson, *Cancer Res.*, **40**, 1699 (1980).

66. G. C. Kennedy, *Proc. Roy. Soc. (London), Ser B*, **140**, 578 (1953).

67. A. Bizzi, S. Garattini, and A. Guiatani, *Europ. J. Cancer*, **4**, 117 (1968).

68. J. J. Kelly and H. A. Waisman, *Blood*, **12**, 635 (1957).

69. C. J. Brackenridge, *Clin. Chim. Acta*, **5**, 539 (1960).

70. P. M. B. Leung, Q. R. Rogers, and A. E. Harper, *J. Nutrition*, **96**, 139 (1968).

71. R. Zender and B. Courvoisier, *Clin. Chim. Acta*, **27**, 259 (1970).

72. Q. R. Rogers and P. M. B. Leung, *Fed. Proc.*, **32**, 1709 (1973).

73. R. Krause, J. H. James, C. Humphrey and J. E. Fischer, *Cancer Res.*, **39**, 3065 (1979).

74. J. D. Radcliffe and S. C. Morrison, *Nutr. Cancer*, **3**, 40 (1981).

75. G. Ollenschlager, R. Lang, W. Feal, and J. Schindler, *Klin. Wochenschr.*, **62**, 1102 (1984).

76. R. W. Begg, *Advan. Cancer Res.*, **5**, 1 (1958).

77. G. Costa, *Rogr. Exp. Tumor Res.*, **3**, 321 (1963).

78. J. P. Mordes, C. Longcope, J. P. Flatt, D. B. MacLean, and A. A. Rossini, *Endocrinology*, **115**, 167 (1984).

79. A. S. Levine and J. E. Morley, *Brain Res.*, **222**, 187 (1981).

80. J. E. Morley and A. S. Levin, *Life Sci.*, **29**, 1901, 1981.

81. S. F. Leibowitz and L. Hor, *Peptides*, **3**, 421 (1982).

82. A. S. Levine, J. Kneip, M. Grace, and J. E. Morley, *Pharmacol. Biochem. Behav.*, **18**, 19 (1983).

83. J. E. Morley, A. S. Levine, G. K. Yim, and M. T. Lowry, *Neurosci. Biobehav. Rev.*, **7**, 281 (1983).

84. G. K. W. Yim and M. T. Lowry, *Fed. Proc.*, **43**, 2893 (1984).

85. L. Grandison and A. Guidotti, *Neuropharmacology*, **16**, 533 (1977).

86. R. Krause, J. H. James, V. Ziparo, and J. E. Fischer, *Cancer*, **44**, 1003 (1979).

87. R. Krause, C. Humphrey, M. Von Meyenfeldt, H. James, and J. E. Fischer, *Cancer Treat. Rep.*, **65**, (Suppl), 15 (1981).

88. M. Von Meyenfeldt, W. T. Chance, and J. F. Fischer, *Am. J. Surg.*, **143**, 133 (1982).

89. W. T. Chance, M. Von Meyenfeldt, and J. E. Fischer, *Pharmacol. Biochem. Behav.*, **17**, 1043 (1982).

90. W. T. Chance, M. VonMeyenfeldt, and J. E. Fischer, *Pharmacol. Biochem. Behav.*, **18**, 115 (1983).

91. W. T. Chance, M. F. Von Meyenfeldt, and J. E. Fischer, *Neurosci. Biobehav. Rev.*, **7**, 471, 1983.

92. M. Nichols, R. P. Maickel, and G. K. W. Yim, *Life Sci.*, **32**, 1819 (1983).

93. M. B. Nichols, R. P. Maickel, and G. K. W. Yim, *Fed. Proc.*, **40**, 256 (1981).

94. M. B. Nichols, R. P. Maickel, and G. K. W. Yim, *Life Sci.*, **36**, 2223 (1985).

95. J. Gibbs, R. C. Young, and G. P. Smith, *J. Comp. Physiol. Psychol.*, **84**, 488 (1973).

96. J. Antin, J. Gibbs, J. Holt, R. C. Young, and G. P. Smith, *J. Comp. Physiol. Psychol.*, **89,** 784 (1975).

97. F. M. Van Lammeren, W. T. Chance, and J. E. Fischer, *Peptides*, **5,** 97 (1984).

98. W. T. Chance, F. M. Van Lammeren, M. E. Chen, W. J. Chen, R. F. Murphy, S. N. Joffe, and J. E. Fischer, *J. Surg. Res.*, **36,** 490 (1984).

99. J. E. Morley, A. S. Levine, G. K. Yim, and M. T. Lowy, *Neurosci. Biobehav. Rev.*, **7,** 281 (1983).

100. B. G. Hoebel, in A. J. Stunkard and E. Stellar, Eds., *Eating and Its Disorders*, Vol. 62, Assoc. Res. Nerv. Med. Disord., Raven Press, New York, 1984, p. 15.

101. B. Barai and W. DeWys, *Proc. Am. Assoc. Cancer Res.*, **21,** 378 (1980).

102. A. Theologides, *Cancer*, **43,** 2004 (1979).

103. F. M. Torti, B. Dieckmann, B. Beutler, A. Cerami, and G. M. Ringold, *Science*, **229,** 867 (1985).

104. B. Beutler, I. W. Milsark, and A. C. Cerami, *Science*, **229,** 869 (1985).

105. A. Theologides, in J. A. Spittell, Ed., *Clinical Medicine*, Lippincott, Philadelphia, 1985 (In press).

106. P. Gallagher and D. E. Tweedle, *J. Par. Enter. Nutr.*, **7,** 361 (1983).

107. G. Hilt and K. A. Bungeroth, *Much. Med. Wochenschr.*, **113,** 91 (1971).

108. G. Irsy and E. Szatloczky, *Ther. Hung.*, **25,** 115 (1977).

109. J. E. Morley, S. D. Morrison, and J. A. Norton, *Cancer Res.*, **45,** 4925 (1985).

110. E. Bruera, E. Roca, L. Cedaro, S. Carraro, and R. Chacon, *Cancer Treat. Rep.*, **69,** 751 (1985).

111. M. Von Meyenfeldt, R. Krause, B. Jeppsson, J. H. James, W. Chance, and J. E. Fischer, *Gastroenterology,* **78** 1286 (1980).

112. J. C. Wallwork, G. J. Fosmire, and H. H. Sandstead, *Br. J. Nutr.*, **45,** 127 (1981).

113. M. B. Essatara, J. E. Morley, A. S. Levine, M. K. Elson, R. B. Shafer, and C. J. McClain, *Physiol. Behav.*, **32,** 475 (1984).

114. V. Voyatzoglou, T. Mountokalakis, V. Tsata-Voyatzoglou, A. Koutselinis, and G. Skalkeas, *Am. J. Surg.*, **144,** 355 (1982).

115. S. Safai-Kutti and J. Kutti, *Ann. Int. Med.*, **100,** 317 (1984).

116. D. Bryce-Smith and R. I. D. Simpson, *Lancet*, **2,** 350 (1984).

9

Appetite Regulation in Anorexia Nervosa

KATHERINE A. HALMI, M.D.
Cornell University Medical College, New York Hospital-Westchester Division,
White Plains, New York

Appetite regulation in anorexia nervosa has not been studied directly. Since the psychological factors of disturbance of body image or disturbance in the way the body is experienced and the fear of getting fat are so prominent in this disorder, which has been regarded as a form of "willful" starvation, the appetite regulation in anorexia nervosa has been ignored. Anorexia nervosa patients when they are not severely emaciated will state that indeed they *do* have an appetite but they refuse to eat because they are afraid they will become fat (1).

Appetite regulation in anorexia nervosa is best examined by studying hunger and satiety phenomena in this disorder. The patterns of eating behavior and weight in anorexia and bulimia nervosa provide a good suspicion for differences in the detection of satiety. There are anorexia nervosa patients who maintain their underweight condition exclusively by restricting food intake. Other anorexia nervosa patients do not have this control and alternate severe food restriction with binge eating. Normal weight bulimia patients have weight fluctuations that are large but are within 10% of normal weight range. In these patients food restriction often alternates with binge eating, or constant binge eating is present with purging behaviors. For some reason these patients are not successful in obtaining and maintaining an *underweight* condition.

Animal studies have shown that during food deprivation there is a decrease of alpha-adrenergic receptor binding in the paraventricular nucleus (PVN). This could mean an increase in the release of PVN-norepinephrine (NE), resulting in receptor down regulation and an inhibition of satiety (2). Increased alpha-adrenergic receptor binding is present in the lateral hypothalamus during food deprivation. This could mean a suppression of NE release here and a receptor proliferation of up regulation to facilitate increased hunger (3). Impairment in the regulation of receptor sites could account for differences in satiety and appetite in normal weight bulimics, underweight anorectics, and underweight anorectics with bulimia.

Appetite regulation could also be reflected in taste hedonics. The hypothalamus may be involved in conditioning mechanisms of taste. Lateral hypothalamic cells alter their rate of firing in response to the taste of a palatable food and fire with a background rate that is correlated with food deprivation (4). Lateral hypothalamic cells can fire during operant barpress responses to obtain food and fire discriminately to food cues (5). Specific neurotransmitter systems can trigger specific appetites. For example, norepinephrine induced feeding is preferential for carbohydrates. Morphine treated rats tend to select fatty foods and naloxone shifts food choice away from fats (6,7).

Anorexia nervosa patients refuse to eat high carbohydrate foods; paradoxically some will binge on high fat and high sugar foods. Taste preferences of restricting anorectics may be a good predictor of bulimic behavior after weight restoration. To study appetite regulation in anorexia nervosa patients we examined the detection of hunger and satiety in these patients in a test meal paradigm.

METHODS

Twelve female anorexia nervosa patients (six were exclusive dieters or restrictors and six had bulimia) and 15 normal female control subjects were studied. Patients were tested upon admission to the inpatient eating disorder unit and again at several weeks after weight restoration. Normal control subjects, from a local college, were tested at similar time intervals. On both testing occasions two pairs of tests were conducted. On one presentation the reservoir of food was hidden from the subject's view and on the other it was uncovered and the patient could view the amount of food she was taking. The order of presentations was randomized for each pair. All patients fasted after midnight until the morning test, which occurred at 10 AM. All patients received chocolate flavored Sustacal, a liquid meal at 1 cal/ml. The subject controlled the rate of intake of food by pressing a button that controlled a small peristaltic pump. The food was delivered to the patient's mouth by a straw. The subject also controlled the length of the meal and told the tester when she was finished. Every two minutes the subject made ratings on visual analog scales for hunger and fullness. These ratings began eight minutes before the meal and continued during the meal and for 14 minutes after completion of the meal.

RESULTS

There were both quantitative and qualitative differences in the hunger and satiety responses between the anorexia nervosa patients and control subjects. The quantitative results are presented in Table 9-1.

Before treatment the anorectic restrictors unexpectedly ate larger meals than the anorectic bulimics and control subjects (mean values = 576 ml, 382 ml, and 281 ml, respectively). After reaching a normal weight, anorectic restrictors tended to eat smaller meals than anorectic bulimics (mean values = 209 ml and 342 ml, respectively).

Before treatment during the course of the meal, anorectic restrictors showed a greater change than anorectic bulimics in both hunger rating (mean values = −41 and −23, respectively) and fullness rating (mean values = +66 and +44, respectively). After reaching a normal weight, anorectic restrictors showed much less change in these ratings than the anorectic bulimics during the meal (anorectic restrictors' hunger change was −23, anorectic bulimics' hunger change was −31). The anorectic restrictors' fullness change after treatment was +18 and the anorectic bulimics' fullness change was +50. After weight restoration there were few dif-

Table 9–1. Hunger and Satiety Responses in a Test Meal

Dx	n	% Target Weight	Test Meal Intake (ml)	Hunger (VAS,mm)			Fullness (VAS,mm)		
				Premeal	Post meal	Change	Premeal	Post meal	Change
				Pretreatment					
AN-R	6	81±6	576±386	57±18	14±16	41±24	16±11	88±10	66±22
AN-B	6	89±8	382±287	64±14	42±32	23±27	23±28	66±25	44±43
				Posttreatment					
AN-R	5	99±1	209±107	55±16	34±11	23±23	25±17	41±26	18±17
AN-B	3	101±2	342±198	64±13	31±7	31±7	22±22	71±11	50±18
Cont.	15	101±12	281±141	52±17	24±28	24±28	24±12	65±19	44±24

ferences between patients and control subjects. The anorectic restrictors had significantly less postmeal fullness and significantly less change in fullness ratings over the meal compared with control subjects ($p < .04$). After treatment the postmeal hunger ratings were significantly greater than the postmeal hunger ratings before treatment ($p < .05$). An increase in weight was the only significant change in the anorectic bulimics over the course of treatment (8).

There was also a qualitative change in the hunger and satiety ratings over treatment and between groups. In the control subjects and in the emaciated anorectic restrictors, the hunger and satiety curves were inversely proportional; however, in the anorectic bulimics there was a rapid rebound of hunger that occurred before the end of the meal and continued after the end of the meal. After weight restoration the anorectic restrictors showed a marked disturbance in hunger and fullness curves. Their curves were no longer reciprocal, as in normal control subjects, and at some points these patients could not distinguish between fullness and hunger, a phenomenon noted consistently in the anorectic bulimic patients (9).

The larger meal taken in the test situation by the anorectic restrictors may reflect their nutritional needs rather than their psychological state. After treatment the anorectic restrictors behaved like restrained eaters in that they ended a meal when they were still hungry and not satiated. The hunger–fullness curves showed distinct differences between the anorectic patients and control subjects, indicating a marked disturbance in the way anorectic patients *experience* hunger and satiety. The continued development of a valid test meal paradigm would allow the specific testing of various neurotransmitter agonists and antagonists relevant to satiety and hunger mechanisms and hence to appetite regulation in anorexia and bulimia nervosa.

At the end of the test meals all subjects answered four satiety questions that were rated on a scale from 1=absent to 5=extreme. These results are presented in Table 9-2.

It is of interest to note that the bulimic anorectics needed significantly more willpower to stop eating in both pretreatment and posttreatment conditions compared to the other groups. The con-

Table 9-2. Appetite and Satiety Questions in Anorexia Nervosa[a]

Urge to Eat	Preoccupation with Food	Willpower to Stop Eating	Satisfaction at End of Meal
		Pretreatment	
AN-R(6)	1.5 ± 0.71	2.2 ± 1.15	1.8 ± 0.76	3.8 ± 0.76
AN-B(6)	2.3 ± 1.13	2.7 ± 1.08	2.6 ± 1.43[b]	3.0 ± 1.09[b]
CONT(15)	1.9 ± 0.51	1.8 ± 0.48	1.5 ± 0.67	2.5 ± 0.74
		Posttreatment	
AN-R(5)	2.0 ± 0.79	1.9 ± 0.75	1.7 ± 0.45	2.1 ± 0.89
AN-B(3)	2.3 ± 1.04	2.33 ± 1.53	2.5 ± 0.87[b]	3.2 ± 0.76
CONT(3)	1.2 ± 0.29	1.0 ± 0	1.17 ± 0.29	3 ± 0

[a]All questions are rated 1 = absent to 5 = extreme.
[b]Analysis of variance, $p. < .05$.

cept of satisfaction after a meal is complicated and it seems contra-
dictory that the patients were more satisfied at the end of the meal
than the control subjects, when the patients had to use greater
willpower to stop eating. It should be noted that the number of
patients in each group being studied, especially during posttreatment, is very small. It is likely when larger numbers are studied
that the trend for anorectic bulimics to have a significantly greater
urge to eat after the meal will be apparent and the trend for the
anorectic bulimics to have a greater preoccupation with food after
the end of the meal will also become significant. Both the satiety
questions and the hunger and fullness profiles during the meal
show the anorectic bulimics to have a more chaotic "psychology"
of hunger and satiety. This is well reflected in their chaotic binge
eating behavior.

It is reasonable to assume that specific taste preferences can
be reflective of appetite regulation based on the studies discussed
earlier (1-7). For example, the specific taste preferences could reflect specific satiety impairments.

METHODS

The subjects tasted 20 chilled (5 cc) mixtures of milk, cream, and
sugar using standard sip and spit procedure. A full factorial design
was used, with four levels of sucrose (0%-20% w/w) and 5 levels of
lipid (0%-25% w/w). Each sample was judged along two, nine-
point adjective scales (sweet and fat) and along a mini-point hedonic preference (dislike–like). The table below is a summary of
the experimental design for 20 taste stimuli.

	Fat per 100g (g)	Sucrose Levels (% Weight/weight)			
Skim milk	0.1	0	5	10	20
Milk	3.5	0	5	10	20
Half and Half	11.7	0	5	10	20
Heavy cream	37.6	0	5	10	20
Cream and oil	52.6	0	5	10	20

The stimuli were presented in a randomized order to reduce potential biases due to the loss of discrimination or taste fatigue. The subjects were instructed to rinse their mouths with water between testing the samples. The patients were tested on admission to the Westchester Division Eating Disorders Program and at the time of discharge about two to three months later.

RESULTS

Two studies have been conducted; the first is presented in Table 9-3. There are significant differences in optimally preferred mixtures of sucrose and lipid between all groups. It is of interest to note that the anorexia nervosa patient had a preference for much lower lipid concentration compared to the other groups and that the obese adults had a very high preference for a high lipid containing solution. Note that the obese adults, on the other hand, had an optimal preference for a very low sucrose concentration and that the highest preferred sucrose concentration was present in the anorexia nervosa patients (10).

In a second study anorectic restrictors, anorectic bulimics, and normal weight bulimic patients were compared in the same taste study before and after weight gain. The population studied is described in Table 9-4 and the results of the testing are listed in Table 9-5.

It is important to note that all patient groups accurately determined the increased concentration of both sweetness and fatiness and were not different from control subjects in their intensity estimates. There were no differences in perception of increasing sweetness or fattiness over treatment. In contrast, *taste preference* varied across subject groups. Bulimic patients gave the greatest pleasantness scores and showed an enhanced liking for intensely sweet (20% sucrose w/w). Exclusive dieting (restrictor) anorectics consistently rated all sucrose and fat stimuli as more unpleasant than bulimics or anorectics with bulimia. These differences were not substantially altered by weight gain during treatment. Taste preferences to sugar and fat appear linked to eating patterns that

Table 9–3. Taste Preferences for Lipid and Sugar as a Function of Body Weight Status

Subject Group	N	Mean Age	Weight (kg)	bmi (wt/ht²)	Optimally Preferred Mixture	
					Sucrose(%)	Lipid(%)
Anorexia nervosa	11	19.3	40.2	15.3	14.9 ± 1.9	12.2 ± 5.1
College students	11	19–21[a]	56.0	20.1	10.4 ± 2.1	22.8 ± 6.3
Adults	15	30.1	58.8	21.6	7.7 ± 1.7	20.7 ± 5.1
Obese adults	12	38.0	95.8	34.4	4.4 ± 1.6	34.1 ± 6.2

[a]Range.

133

Table 9–4. Characteristics of Eating Disorder Patients

Diagnosis	Age (yrs)	Weight (kg) Pre-	Weight (kg) Post-
Anorexia restrictor (n = 5)	16.0 + 0.9	38.0 + 1.7	48.3 + 1.7
Anorexia with bulimia (n = 11)	19.6 + 1.3	43.9 + 2.3	50.5 + 1.4
Bulimia (n = 4)	19.2 + 1.7	52.9 + 2.1	55.0 + 1.6

define the eating disorder groups and thus may provide a psycho-
biological marker of a psychiatric diagnosis (11). Specific pharmacologic interventions to treat bulimic behavior may well affect
taste preference, and a measure of taste preferences could well be
a predictor for treatment outcome.

In one study examining the treatment efficacy of the antihista-
mine cyproheptadine and the antidepressant amitriptyline in the
treatment of anorexia nervosa, there was a surprising differential
drug effect present on the bulimic anorectic patients. Cyprohep-

**Table 9–5. Intensity Estimates and Preference Ratings
of Taste Testing**

Intensity Estimates	F Values	Significance
Sweet		
Main effect of sugar	$F(3,63)$ = 184.86	$p < .01$
Main effect of fat	$F(4,84)$ = 12.99	$p < .01$
Fat × sugar interaction	$F(12,252) =$ 2.05	$p < .05$
Fat		
Main effect of fat	$F(4,84)$ = 70.20	$p < .01$

Preference Ratings	F Values	Significance
Main effect of group	$F(2,17) = 3.93$	$p < .05$
Main effect of sugar	$F(3,51) = 9.95$	$p < .01$
Main effect of fat	$F(4,69) = 5.74$	$p < .01$

tadine, which is a serotonin antagonist, significantly decreased treatment efficiency (rate of weight gain) for the anorectic bulimic patients when compared to the amitriptyline and placebo groups (12). It seems reasonable to postulate that cyproheptadine is having a differential effect on appetite regulation as reflected in eating behavior and weight gain in the anorectic bulimic patients.

The study of appetite regulation in anorexia nervosa has been ignored until recently. It is possible that the prolonged periods of severe dieting can have a permanent effect on appetite regulation in anorexia nervosa. This may explain the very high incidence of bulimia that develops in weight restored anorexia nervosa patients. To develop more effective treatment programs for anorexia nervosa patients as well as to continue to study basic mechanisms of appetite regulation, it is important to continue to develop creative and systematic, methodologically sound investigations of hunger and satiety in the eating disorder patients.

REFERENCES

1. K. A. Halmi, *Comprehensive Textbook of Psychiatry,* 4th Ed., Volume 2, Williams and Wilkins, Baltimore/London, 1985, pp. 1143–48.

2. B. Hoebel, *Eating and Its Disorders,* Raven Press, New York, 1984, pp. 15–38.

3. M. Jhanwar-Uniyal, F. Fleischer, and B. E. Levine, *Abstract Soc. Neuroscience,* **8,** 711 (1982).

4. E. T. Rolls, *The Neural Basis of Feeding and Reward,* Haer Institute, Brunswick, Maine, 1982, p. 323.

5. H. Nishino, *The Neural Basis of Feeding and Reward,* Haer Institute, Brunswick, Maine, 1982, pp. 355–372.

6. S. F. Leibowitz, *Handbook of Hypothalamus,* Vol. 3, 1982, pp. 299–437.

7. R. Marx-Kaufman and R. B. Kamarek, *Psychopharmacology,* **74,** 321 (1981).

8. K. A. Halmi, W. P. Owen, J. Gibbs, and G. Smith, presented at the International Meeting of Biological Psychiatry, Philadelphia, PA, September 10, 1985.

9. W. P. Owen, K. A. Halmi, J. Gibbs, and G. Smith, *J. Psychiat. Res.,* **19,** 279 (1985).

10. A. Drewnowski, M. R. C. Greenwood, K. A. Halmi, J. Gibbs, and P. Duberstein, *Fed. Proc.,* **43,** 475, (1984).

11. K. A. Halmi, A. Drewnowski, B. Pierce, J. Gibbs, and G. P. Smith, *APA Syllabus and Proceedings,* 1985, p. 81.

12. K. A. Halmi, E. Eckert, T. J. LaDu, and J. Cohen, *Arch. Gen. Psychiat.,* in press.

10

Appetite Regulation in Bulimia

B. TIMOTHY WALSH, M.D.
College of Physicians & Surgeons, Columbia University, New York, New York

Bulimia is an eating disorder whose salient characteristic is episodic binge eating. Patients with bulimia are aware that the behavior is abnormal but feel unable to control their eating during a binge. Most patients with bulimia attempt to avoid weight gain by inducing vomiting after binges, by abusing laxatives or diuretics, or by severely restricting their diets between binges. Bulimia can occur at both ends of the weight spectrum; about one-half of patients hospitalized for anorexia nervosa also binge eat, so they can be considered to have both anorexia nervosa and bulimia (1,2). Conversely, a fraction of overweight patients also engages in binge eating behavior (3,4). However, the majority of patients who present themselves to clinics requesting treatment for bulimia are of normal body weight (5). In such patients, the frequency of binges ranges from a few times a month to five or more episodes a day, and the average amount of food consumed per binge is several thousand calories.

Although this pattern of eating was described in antiquity, bulimia attracted little medical attention until the late 1970s. Since that time, there has been a flurry of popular and professional interest in this syndrome. Despite stories in newspapers and magazines suggesting that bulimia is epidemic, we have few accurate estimates of its frequency in the general population. Surveys of selected populations, typically female college students, suggest

This work was supported in part by Grants MH-38355 and MH-00383 from NIMH.

that loosely defined "binge eating" is a common occurrence. When more restrictive criteria are applied, such as a minimum binge frequency of once a week and the routine use of purging, estimates of the frequency of bulimia drop considerably, but are still in the range of 1% to 5% of young women, a disturbingly high prevalence (6–10).

In normal weight individuals, bulimia appears to be generally well tolerated physically. The disturbances most frequently noted are fluid and electrolyte abnormalities related to recurrent vomiting or laxative and diuretic abuse or both (11). These metabolic derangements can produce physical symptoms and are occasionally of sufficient severity to require acute medical intervention. Gastric dilatation and rupture, which are life-threatening complications, have rarely been reported (12,13). Patients who induce vomiting may develop significant dental disease, probably related to the effects of stomach acid on the teeth, and painless, benign salivary gland enlargement (14–16). Women with bulimia also appear to have a higher than expected frequency of menstrual disturbance.

In trying to understand the characteristics of the syndrome of bulimia, it is important to note that it appears to be related to the syndrome of anorexia nervosa. As already noted, about one-half of patients hospitalized for anorexia nervosa also have the behavioral pattern of bulimia. And, about one-third of patients who present themselves to clinics for treatment of bulimia, although they are of normal weight when they request treatment, have past histories of anorexia nervosa. Thus, both anorexia nervosa and bulimia appear to be illnesses that primarily affect young adult women in this culture, and also appear to be illnesses with a significant overlap in symptomatology and in clinical course.

EATING BEHAVIOR IN BULIMIA

We have very little knowledge about appetite regulation in patients with bulimia. In fact, we know little about what such patients eat, much less about the factors that influence their eating. In devising hypotheses about the regulation of appetite in patients with binge eating, it is important, if not necessary, to know what the behavior is for which we must account.

The common clinical impression is that patients binge on foods high in carbohydrates, and that they tend to diet between binges. A few investigations have attempted to assess the dietary patterns of patients with bulimia when they are not bingeing. Weiss and Ebert (17) obtained information on dietary habits from interviews with 15 women of normal weight with bulimia and 15 age- and sex-matched control subjects. Compared to the control subjects, the patients reported that they fasted more frequently, that they more frequently abstained from food while hungry, and that they ate fewer times per day (2.9 vs. 4.6). Ten of the 15 bulimic patients tried to limit scheduled meals to low calorie foods, while control subjects ate a greater variety. Similarly, Mitchell and colleagues (5) reported that only 21% of 256 bulimic patients said that they ate two or more normal meals a day, while 21% indicated they ate normal meals less than once a week or not at all.

Mitchell and Laine (18) have recently reported the results of a study in which six normal weight bulimic women were permitted to follow their usual patterns of eating during a 24 hour period of hospitalization. In their nonbinge meals during that day, the subjects consumed an average of only 451 calories (range 69 to 1,062 calories). Rosen and colleagues (19) asked 20 patients with bulimia and 20 control subjects to eat as much of a large meal as they comfortably could. The patients consumed on average 27% of the meal, compared to 70% consumed by the control subjects. These limited data are consistent with the clinical impression that not only the binge eating behavior but also the nonbinge eating behavior of patients with bulimia is disturbed. Specifically, these patients appear to eat fewer meals and fewer calories in nonbinge situations than their peers.

A few data are also available concerning the nutritional content of foods consumed during a binge. Mitchell and colleagues (20) obtained records from 25 patients in which they recorded what they consumed during a binge. The foods tended to be those high in both carbohydrates and fat, such as ice cream, and the mean number of calories per binge was 3,415. However, there was a large range in the reported contents of binges, from a low of 1,200 calories to a high of 11,500 calories per binge. Likewise, Abraham and Beumont (21) report that bulimic patients' records of foods consumed during a binge suggest that the nutritional content of a binge is quite variable.

Two groups have reported data from patients' bingeing in the laboratory. In the study of Mitchell and Laine (18) mentioned above, six bulimic women were permitted to binge eat in the hospital for 24 hours. They were provided by the hospital with the foods that they specified as being ones they would wish to eat during a binge. The subjects were not directly observed while eating, but were instructed to signal the nursing staff when they were about to binge eat, and after they had completed a binge. The mean number of calories consumed per binge eating episode was 4,394 but with a range of 1,436 to 8,585 calories. The average nutritional content was 49% carbohydrate, 43% fat, and 8% protein, although this varied substantially as well, ranging from 31% to 58% carbohydrate, from 34% to 50% fat, and from 4% to 19% protein.

Kaye and his co-workers at NIMH (22) have conducted a similar experiment in 12 normal weight women with bulimia. The mean content of a binge was 3,500 calories (range 1,570 to 6,370). The nutritional content of the binge was carbohydrate 52% (range 37% to 76%), fat 37% (range 14% to 46%), and protein 11.2% (range 8% to 17%).

In collaboration with Drs. Harry Kissileff, John Kral, and their colleagues at St. Lukes-Roosevelt Hospital, we have recently conducted some preliminary studies of the eating behavior of bulimic patients in a laboratory setting. Our results, although from only seven patients, appear to confirm and to extend the studies of Mitchell and Laine, and of Kaye and colleagues. Our protocol differs from those already described in several ways. Patients were, on two occasions, invited to eat a "meal" alone in a room. Each patient was provided, on both occasions, with the same variety of foods, which included vegetables, meat, bread, salad, and ice cream. On one occasion, the patients were asked to "let yourself go and to overeat." On the other occasion, the patients were asked to eat what they would "normally consume in a relaxed atmosphere." Thus, we have been attempting to assess both binge eating and normal eating under relatively standardized conditions.

When the patients were asked to overeat, they consumed an average of 3,630 calories (range 2,083 to 8,499), consisting of 47.5% carbohydrates (range 43% to 50%), 39.5% fat (range 35% to 43%), and 13.1% protein (range 8% to 22%). These results are reassuringly similar to those of Mitchell and Laine, and of Kaye and colleagues (18,22).

Five of the seven patients, although asked to eat a "normal" meal, were unable to control their eating under these circumstances, and binged, consuming, on average, 3,442 calories. The two patients who did not binge consumed only 283 calories. These preliminary data seem to us to support two clinical impressions concerning patients with bulimia, namely that their nonbinge meals are relatively low in calories, and that they have great difficulty controlling their eating when given access to a large amount of food.

In summary, although the data are meager, the descriptions of the eating behavior of patients with bulimia are fairly consistent. Specifically, the characteristics of eating behavior in bulimia include the following:

1. Patients with this illness do, indeed, during a binge, consume several thousands of calories in less than one hour.

2. The nutritional content of a binge tends to be high in carbohydrate and high in fat; however, in this respect the nutritional content of a binge closely resembles the nutritional content of freely selected human diets (23).

3. There is substantial variation among patients both in calories consumed and in the nutritional content of a binge.

4. Patients with bulimia "normally" appear to eat few calories per nonbinge meal, and have significant difficulty preventing a normal meal from developing into a binge.

At present, we do not have a comprehensive model of eating behavior in bulimia that accounts for all of these clinical phenomena. Rather, several different and for the most part complementary hypotheses have been suggested, which attempt to account for certain aspects of the syndrome. In the remainder of this chapter, I will provide a brief summary of some of these hypotheses.

DIETARY DEPRIVATION

One line of thought about the eating behavior of patients with bulimia is based on the clinical impression, supported, as described above, by a small amount of experimental data, that patients with bulimia restrict their caloric intake between binges. That is, they are imposing on themselves transient episodes of caloric deprivation.

A second reason for suspecting that caloric deprivation may play a role in the development and perpetuation of bulimia is the fact that many patients of normal body weight with bulimia give histories that are suggestive of a disturbance of body weight. Russell (24) in his description of the syndrome of bulimia nervosa in 30 patients, noted that the average patient was 7 kg below her premorbid weight and "struggling" to avoid gaining weight. Abraham and Beumont (21) described an impressive degree of weight fluctuation among 32 patients with bulimia, and noted that one-half of the patients were attempting to maintain themselves at weights lower than those at which they had previously been stable. Similarly, Fairburn and Cooper (25) found that 43% of a series of 35 patients with bulimia had once weighed more than 120% of the matched population mean weight, compared to less than 6% at the time of presentation. Mitchell and colleagues (5) found that 56% of 275 patients had, since age 18, weighed at least 10% over ideal body weight compared to only 20% of the 275 patients at the time of presentation. Thus, it is common for bulimic patients to have past histories of mild obesity and it is characteristic of such patients to be maintaining a lower than premorbid weight.

The role of caloric deprivation in the initiation of the syndrome of bulimia is also suggested by the frequency with which patients report that their bulimic behavior began at a time that they were dieting. In a description of 34 patients of normal weight with bulimia, Pyle and colleagues (26) found that, in 30, the bulimia had begun during a period of voluntary dieting. A similar observation was made by Abraham and Beumont (21). Thus, patients of normal weight with bulimia often begin to binge eat during a diet, many attempt to maintain weights that are lower than their premorbid weights, and, from the limited amount of data avilable, appear to be on restricted diets when they are not bingeing.

How might this caloric deprivation be related to binge eating? A major source of data about the behavioral effects of caloric deprivation on subsequent eating behavior is the remarkable series of experiments conducted during World War II at the University of Minnesota (27). Thirty-six normal young men who were conscientious objectors volunteered to submit themselves to a semistarvation diet. For three months, observations were made while the patients received a weight maintenance diet of approximately 3,500 calories per day. Then the men were placed on a semistarvation diet containing 1,570 calories per day. During the six month period of semistarvation, the average weight loss was 24% of the control value. The observations of the men during this six month period of semistarvation are a rich source of information on the effects of caloric deprivation on a group of people who were both relatively normal before the beginning of the experiment and who were not subjected to the traumatic effects of war, imprisonment, torture, or gross famine, which are usually responsible for severe caloric deprivation. The semistarvation period was followed by three months of controlled rehabilitation, during which the caloric allotment was slowly increased, but at the end of this period, the men were still significantly undernourished. When the men were finally given free access to food, they appeared to have serious difficulty controlling themselves (28). They are reported to have "gorged prodigious quantities of food, which approximated 6,000 to 7,000 calories per day." One of the men became acutely ill because of overeating and required hospitalization for a week.

These data suggest that severe caloric deprivation followed by access to food produces binge eating behavior very similar to that of bulimic patients even in individuals who had previously had no eating disorder. It should be emphasized that most patients with bulimia have never experienced the degree of starvation produced by the experiments at the University of Minnesota. However, the data do suggest that a contributing factor to binge eating may be caloric deprivation. Thus, the constant dieting of the patients with bulimia may be one factor that helps perpetuate the pathologic behavior.

These observations lead to several hypotheses about the role of dietary deprivation in the behavioral abnormalities of bulimia. Polivy and Herman (29), extending their work on restrained eaters, have argued that dieting causes bingeing by promoting the adoption of a cognitively regulated eating style. To maintain weight loss individuals who binge eat adopt a rigid cognitive stance that overrides physiological cues. A variety of experiences, such as anxiety, alcohol, or the impression that they have broken their diet, may lead to disinhibition of the cognitive controls, and, thus, to an episode of bingeing. Although most of the experimental work in this area has been carried out in restrained eaters who did not have bulimia, it appears that, as suggested by Polivy and Herman, most patients with bulimia would be classified as restrained eaters, and that a variety of "triggers" can lead to binge eating. A number of other investigators (30,31) have emphasized the role of cognitive factors in the development of inappropriately severe dieting and have developed treatment programs that focus on these disturbed cognitions.

A complementary hypothesis based on the presence of dietary deprivation is that significant physiologic factors predispose patients with bulimia to binge eat. For example, it can be argued that many patients with bulimia are attempting to maintain body weights below their physiologic "set points" and that they are being biologically driven to overeat in order to restore their weights to the appropriate levels. This model does not really demand the existence of a biologically determined set point, but does assume that physiologic drives to eat are somehow activated or increased after a certain amount of weight loss (32). While this model is heuristically appealing, it is limited by the absence of any objective means of assessing these physiologic drives. Despite this caveat, it would be of interest to determine if patients of normal body weight with bulimia exhibit any of the physiologic alterations suggested by some studies to occur in obese individuals who have lost weight, such as reduced fat cell size, increased adipose tissue lipoprotein lipase activity, and reduced diet induced thermogenesis (33,34).

Even if we cannot reliably determine, at present, whether patients with bulimia are below their physiologic set points, we can ask if they show any physiologic evidence of caloric deprivation. Pirke and colleagues (35) recently reported that normal weight patients with bulimia do indeed show metabolic evidence of semistarvation. Specifically, 15 patients with bulimia showed elevated plasma levels of free fatty acids and beta-hydroxybutyric acid, and diminished serum levels of tri-iodothyronine. These data, although preliminary, are consistent with the notion that the weight loss or the restrictive dieting, or both, of many patients with bulimia may lead to physiological aberrations, which, in turn, may be associated with increased appetite.

EMOTIONAL FACTORS

A second line of thinking about appetite regulation in patients with bulimia focuses not on their cognitive or physiologic states, but on their emotional states. There is general agreement among clinicians working with patients with bulimia that compared to their peers, such patients are more anxious, depressed, and irritable. Furthermore, they appear more prone to develop psychiatric syndromes, especially depression (36,37). It is far less clear what is the cart and what is the horse. That is, to what degree are patients with bulimia depressed because they are bingeing, and to what degree are they bingeing because they are depressed? While this issue remains controversial, the observation of the increased frequency of mood disturbance among these patients appears generally accepted, and leads to at least two types of hypotheses about appetite regulation.

One hypothesis is that increased appetite, carbohydrate craving, and binge eating are manifestations of a depressive syndrome. Disturbances of appetite are common in patients with significant depression. While loss of appetite is a criterion for classic, melancholic depression, an increase in appetite and, specifically, in carbohydrate craving, has been described as characteristic of other depressive syndromes, such as "atypical" depression and seasonal affective disorder (38,39). Thus, some patients with bulimia may be suffering from a depressive syndrome manifested, in part, by binge eating. A piece of evidence often cited to support this model is the apparent utility of antidepressant medication in bulimia (40–42). But, we should be very cautious about drawing etiological conclusions from treatment studies. Simply because a medication used to treat depression relieves an illness does not conclusively prove that the illness was depression. (A similar caveat can be applied to the results of any treatment study.) There is currently significant controversy about the degree of symptomatic, familial, and biological similarity between the depression in bulimia and that in typical major affective illness, and it is possible that we must await a reliable, independent "marker" for major affective illness before being able to determine how many patients with bulimia have an unusual presentation of a typical mood disturbance.

A somewhat different hypothesis involving mood disturbance and bulimia is that patients use binge eating to modulate their moods. A number of investigators have noted that dysphoric emotional states, particularly anxiety, are the most frequent precipitants of binge eating, and that there is at least a transient reduction in anxiety after the binge has concluded (5,21,43). Conceivably, diet induced alterations in CNS neurotransmitter concentrations may contribute to changes in mood after binge eating (44). Thus, binge eating may be perpetuated by patients' using the behavior to modulate unpleasant affective states. This hypothesis suggests that bulimia is linked to a wider range of emotions than just depression, and provides a rationale for the clinical similarities between bulimia and addictive disorders.

A variant of this hypothesis is that of Rosen and Leitenberg (45), who have suggested that the critical element in the reduction of anxiety after binge eating is self induced vomiting. Their group has described the successful treatment of bulimia by using exposure (i.e., eating feared foods) plus response prevention (i.e., vomiting). Although this hypothesis focuses attention on an important element of the syndrome and may suggest an effective treatment modality, it does not provide a satisfying explanation of the binge eating itself.

Even this brief and incomplete review illustrates the present diversity of hypotheses concerning the regulation of eating behavior and of appetite in the syndrome of bulimia. I suspect that several factors are responsible for this diversity. First, it is a reflection of our ignorance. Studies of the eating behavior of patients with bulimia have only recently begun, and, until we know more clearly what the phenomena are, it will be difficult to decide among various hypotheses to explain them. Second, the few data that we do have about eating behavior in bulimia suggest that bulimia is both complex and heterogeneous. It seems likely that bulimia is the result of interactions between psychological, physiologic, and nutritional variables, and that there is substantial variability among patients. Different hypotheses may be required to account for various aspects of the syndrome. Last, it seems likely that different factors are important at different stages in the development of bulimia. Weiner (46) has suggested that, in developing an understanding of psychosomatic illnesses, it is important to separate predisposing, initiating, and perpetuating factors and mechanisms. One can conceive, for example, that the current cultural emphasis on thinness predisposes women to diet, that in certain individuals with familial obesity, significant physiologic disturbances develop during the course of dieting which lead to the initiation of bingeing, and that the illness persists because individuals susceptible to depression or anxiety discover they can use binge eating to modulate their mood states. In developing and testing hypotheses about the regulation of appetite in bulimia, it will be important to keep this complexity in mind and to focus experimentally on specific facets and phases of the syndrome.

REFERENCES

1. R. C. Casper, E. D. Eckert, K. A. Halmi, S. C. Goldberg, and J. M. Davis, *Arch. Gen. Psychiat.*, **37,** 1030 (1980).

2. P. E. Garfinkel, H. Moldofsky, and D. M. Garner, *Arch. Gen. Psychiat.*, **37,** 1036 (1980).

3. A. J. Stunkard, *Psychiat. Quart.*, **33,** 284 (1959).

4. J. Gormally, S. Black, S. Daston, and D. Rardin, *Addictive Behav.*, **7,** 47 (1982).

5. J. E. Mitchell, D. Katsukami, E. D. Eckert, and R. L. Pyle, *Am. J. Psychiat.*, **142,** 482 (1985).

6. K. A. Halmi, J. R. Falk, and E. Schwartz, *Psychol. Med.*, **11**, 697 (1981).

7. R. L. Pyle, J. E. Mitchell, E. D. Eckert, P. A. Halvorson, P. A. Neuman, and G. Goff, *Int. J. Eating Disorders*, **2**, 75 (1983).

8. H. G. Pope, J. I. Hudson, and D. Yurgelun-Todd, *Am. J. Psychiat.*, **141**, 292 (1984).

9. P. J. Cooper, G. Waterman, and C. Fairburn, *Br. J. Clin. Psychol.*, **23**, 45 (1984).

10. K. J. Hart and T. H. Ollendick, *Am. J. Psychiat.*, **142**, 851 (1985).

11. J. E. Mitchell, R. L. Pyle, E. D. Eckert, D. Katsukami, and R. Lentz, *Psychol. Med.*, **13**, 272 (1983).

12. M. Matikainen, *Am. J. Surg.*, **138**, 451 (1979).

13. P. G. Devitt and G. W. H. Stamp, *Gut*, **24**, 678 (1983).

14. P. A. Levin, J. M. Falko, K. Dixon, E. M. Gallup, and W. Saunders, *Ann. Int. Med.*, **93**, 827 (1980).

15. B. T. Walsh, C. B. Croft, and J. L. Katz, *Int. J. Psychiat. Med.*, **11**, 255 (1981–2).

16. J. L. Harrison, L. A. George, J. L. Cheatham, and J. Zinn, *Dentistry*, **88**, 65 (1985).

17. S. R. Weiss and M. H. Ebert, *Psychom. Med.*, **45**, 293 (1983).

18. J. E. Mitchell and D. C. Laine, *Int. J. Eating Disorders*, **4**, 177 (1985).

19. J. C. Rosen, H. Leitenberg, K. M. Fondacara, J. Gross, and M. Willmuth, *Int. J. Eating Disorders*, **4**, 59 (1985).

20. J. E. Mitchell, R. L. Pyle, and E. D. Eckert, *Am J. Psychiat.*, **138**, 835 (1981).

21. S. F. Abraham and P. J. V. Beumont, *Psychol. Med.*, **12**, (1982).

22. W. H. Kaye, H. Gwirtsman, T. George, S. R. Weiss, and D. C. Jimerson, Relationship of Mood Alterations to Bingeing Behavior in Bulimia, *Br. J. Psychiat.*, in press.

23. H. R. Kissileff and T. B. Van Itallie, *Ann. Rev. Nutr.*, **2**, 371 (1982).

24. G. Russell, *Psychol. Med.*, **9**, 429 (1979).

25. C. G. Fairburn and P. J. Cooper, *Br. J. Psychiat.*, **144**, 238 (1984).

26. R. L. Pyle, J. E. Mitchell, and E. D. Eckert, *J. Clin. Psychiat.*, **42**, 60 (1981).

27. A. Keys, J. Brozek, A. Henschel, O. Mickelsen, and H. L. Taylor, *The Biology of Human Starvation*, University of Minnesota Press, Minneapolis, 1950.

28. J. C. Franklin, B. C. Schiele, J. Brozek, and A. Keys, *J. Clin. Psychol.*, **4**, 28 (1948).

29. J. Polivy and C. P. Herman, *Am. Psychologist*, **40**, 192 (1985).

30. C. G. Fairburn, "Cognitive-Behavioral Treatment for Bulimia," in D. M. Garner and P. E. Garfinkel, Eds., *Handbook of Psychotherapy for Anorexia Nervosa and Bulimia*, Guilford Press, New York, 1985, pp. 160–192.

31. G. T. Wilson, E. Rossiter, E. Kleifield, and L. Lindholm, Cognitive-Behavioral Treatment of Bulimia Nervosa, *Behavior Research and Therapy*, in press.

32. D. Wirtshafter and J. D. Davis, *Physiol. and Behav.*, **19**, 75 (1977).

33. R. S. Schwartz and J. D. Brunzell, *Lancet*, **1**, 1230 (1978).

34. Y. Schutz, T. Bessard, and J. Jequier, *Am. J. Clin. Nutr.*, **40**, 542 (1984).

35. K. M. Pirke, J. Pahl, U. Schweiger, and M. Warnhoff, *Psychiat. Res.*, **15**, 33 (1985).

36. J. I. Hudson, H. G. Pope, J. M. Jonas, and D. Yurgelun-Todd, *Psychiat. Res.*, **9**, 345 (1983).

37. B. T. Walsh, S. P. Roose, A. H. Glassman, M. Gladis, and C. Sadik, *Psychosom. Med.*, **47**, 123 (1985).

38. J. R. T. Davidson, R. D. Miller, C. D. Turnbull, and J. L. Sullivan, *Arch. Gen. Psychiat.*, **39**, 527–534 (1982).

39. N. E. Rosenthal, D. A. Sack, J. C. Gillin, A. J. Lewy, F. K. Goodwin, Y. Davenport, P. S. Mueller, D. A. Newsome, and T. A. Wehr, *Arch. Gen. Psychiat.*, **41**, 72 (1984).

40. H. G. Pope, J. I. Hudson, J. M. Jonas, and D. Yurgelun-Todd, *Am. J. Psychiat.*, **140**, 554 (1983).

41. B. T. Walsh, J. W. Stewart, S. P. Roose, M. Gladis, and H. Glassman, *Arch. Gen. Psychiat.*, **41**, 1105 (1984).

42. P. L. Hughes, L. A. Wells, and J. C. Cunningham, Presented at the 137th Annual Meeting, American Psychiatric Association, May, 1984.

43. C. Johnson and R. Larson, *Psychom. Med.*, **44**, 341 (1982).

44. R. J. Wurtman, *Lancet*, **1**, 1145 (1983).

45. J. C. Rosen, and H. Leitenberg, "Exposure Plus Response Prevention Treatment of Bulimia," in D. M. Garner and P. E. Garfinkel, Eds., *Handbook of Psychotherapy for Anorexia Nervosa and Bulimia*, Guilford Press, New York, 1985, pp. 193–212.

46. H. Weiner, *Psychobiology and Human Disease*, Elsevier, New York, 1977.

Index

DATE DUE

AUG 0 6 1990		
NOV 0 7 1990		
NOV 1 2 1992		
FEB 2 5 1993		
MAR 1 1 1993		
NOV 2 9 1993		
JUN 2 2 1994		
APR 1 9 1994		
APR 0 1 1998		
APR 1 5 1998		
GAYLORD		PRINTED IN U.S.A.

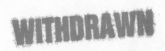